CONTENTS

INTRODUCTION
BAKING BASICS-

Baking required no introduction. It is one of the oldest and most popular cooking methods known to mankind. These days, pretty much every kitchen has the food ingredients and equipment required to bake some delicious goodies.

Baking is a fairly simple process that can be used to prepare food ranging from simple breads to spectacular confectionery.

Before we jump into the recipes, let us take a look at the ingredients and equipment you will need. If you're a veteran baker already, feel free to jump straight into the recipes. If you're a newbie, stick around for a while longer.

Ingredients

In this section we will discuss a few of the most commonly used ingredients in baking recipes.

BUTTER

Butter has an amazing flavour and texture by itself, and when used in baking recipes, it greatly enhances the flavour and texture of the final product. Unsalted butter is best as it gives you full control over the taste of your recipes.

MILK

Milk is one of the most important ingredients when it comes to baking. It makes the four tender, and also forms the base for quite a few recipes.

FLOUR

Always sift the flour before you use in a baking recipe. Pretty much every kind of flour out there can be used for baking, but the most popular kind used for making is "All Purpose Flour". It is easily available, doesn't cost much, and easy to work with.

"Cake Flour" is another kind of flour that is smoother than all purpose flour. It is great for making cake sponges and other tender & spongy baked recipes.

"Pastry Flour" is another flour which works pretty much like cake flour.

"Self-Rising Flour" is basically all-purpose flour mixed with baking powder. To make your own, mix one teaspoon of baking powder for each cup of flour.

"Rye Flour" is a healthy flour with great nutritional benefits. However, it doesn't form gluten strands, making it ill-suited for yeasted dough.

"Oat Flour" is loaded with fiber and protein. It is commonly used in healthy baking recipes.

Almond flour, coconut flour, tapioca flour are a few other flours that are used in baking recipes today.

BAKING POWDER

Baking powder is basically a mixture of baking soda and an acidic component. It is a leavening agent on its own, and doesn't require addition of an acidic ingredient to do its work.

Hundreds of branks make baking powder, and they are all pretty much the same. Just make sure the baking powder you buy is free of aluminium. Baking powder has a shelf life of about six months, so make sure you use it all before that.

BAKING SODA

Baking soda is a leavening agent that requires another acidic ingredient to do its job. It can be stored safely for years.

YEAST

Found commonly in bread, dinner rolls and similar pastries, yeast is a natural leavening agent which does its job by fermenting in the batter or dough, causing a rise in volume by absorbing air.

SUGAR

Excess of sugar leads to a spike in blood glycogen levels, and is rightly blamed for many health problems. Eat sugary delights in moderation, and as a side to a healthy balanced diet. Sugar adds texture, sweetness, and moisture to baked recipes, making it an important ingredient in some of the sweet baked goodies. It promotes the growth of yeast in a few of the recipes too.

There are many kinds of sugars available out there, and every recipe will specify the kind of sugar used. If not mentioned, use the regular granulated sugar. Brown sugar is unrefined white sugar, and has a strong taste of its own, making it unsuitable most of the recipes. However, in some recipes, the flavour of brown sugar compliments the flavour of the recipe.

CHOCOLATE

If a recipe in this book calls for dark chocolate, it is best to use a chocolate that has a cocoa content higher than 70%. Dark chocolate is the most commonly used chocolate in this book, as it has low sugar content, and has a strong flavour and great texture. If a recipe calls for chocolate chips, and you don't have those on hand, just chop up a chunk of dark chocolate into small bits and you're good to go!

White and milk chocolates are quite popular too these days, and taste great due to the high sugar content.

COCOA POWDER

Today, two kinds of cocoa powers are popular- natural cocoa powder, and Dutch processed cocoa powder.

Unless stated otherwise, all cocoa powder used in this book is Dutch processed cocoa powder due to its darker colour and intense taste.

EGGS

Free ranch fresh eggs are best. Unless stated otherwise, all eggs used in this book are medium-sized.

Eggs are one of the most commonly used ingredients in baking as they greatly enhance the texture of cakes and cookies, and allow air to be absorbed into the batter, making it fluffy. They are also help keep the recipes moist.

Eggs are delicious and nutritious on their own, and when used in baking recipes, impart their nutrition, taste, and colour to the recipes.

GELATIN

Gelatin or gelatine is a translucent, colorless, flavorless food ingredient, derived from collagen extracted from animal body parts. It is brittle when dry and gummy when moist. It is used to to stabilize creams or jellies and it needs to be bloomed before use. If you boil it, it loses its strength, so don't do that.

Unless stated otherwise, all gelatin used in this book is powdered or granulated. Leafed gelatin comes in handy sometimes too.

NUTS

Nuts are rich in healthy fats, and taste absolutely scrumptious on pretty much everything baked. Some of the most commonly used nuts in baked recipes are: almonds, coconut, hazelnuts, pecans, peanuts, walnuts, pistachio, macadamia nuts, cashew nuts, etc. Nuts are best used fresh.

SALT

Salt is a common ingredient in all kinds of cooking, and baking is no exception. Salt strengthens the gluten structure, enhances the flavour, and highly useful with yeast.

SPICES

Spices are delicious and nutritious, and add a variety of flavours to baked recipes. One of the most commonly used spices in baking is vanilla. A natural extract of vanilla is best. Cinnamon, ginger, nutmeg, cardamom, orange zest, lemon zest, cloves, lavender, etc are some other spices commonly used in baking.

Equipment

Some cheap basic equipment is all you really need to start baking. You probably already have most of the stuff I am about to list.

BAKING PANS

Small pans, large pans, they all get the job done. Just make sure you have some.

Cake pans are great for making cakes. If you don't intend to make multiple cakes simultaneously, just one pan is all you really need. A basic pan with a diameter of eight to nine inches usually gets the job done. They are easily available in stores, and on amazon.

Bundt cake pans are used to give spectacular shapes to your cakes. They come in pretty much all shapes, sizes, and patterns. Just remember that the more complex the design gets, the harder they are to clean.

Muffin tins are really useful for making muffins, and are easily available on amazon, and in stores around you. I personally prefer muffin tins with **minimum** 12 cups, as I have a family of 4, and 12 cups hits the spot. If you get a smaller one, just reduce the amount of ingredients you use proportionally.

Pie and tart pans are also handy little pans, and it is a good idea to have **minimum** one of each if you wish to make these recipes.

MIXER

You can do all the mixing you will need using your hand and a spoon or whisk, but having a mixer sure makes the job easier. Any old small mixer will do. But then again, it is really not necessary if you don't mind some manual stirring and whisking.

WHISK

Whisks are indispensable tools when it comes to baking. There are manual and electronic whisks easily available today, and they will both get the job done.

SPATULAS AND WOODEN SPOONS

Some mixtures need to be blended slowly to prevent gluten strands from forming, and that is why it is always a good idea to keep spatulas and wooden spoons handy.

FOOD PROCESSOR

Food processors are cheap, and can make certain grinding tasks a piece of cake!

MEASURING SPOONS AND CUPS

You will need some a few measuring instruments as all recipes call for specific quantities of ingredients. If you're a veteran cook, you're probably good at approximation by now, but measuring instruments are indispensable for the newbies.

American measuring sets are quite cheap, and one set contains all standard measurements used in this book, so go grab a set if you don't have one already.

MIXING BOWLS

Steel and glass mixing containers are my favourite.

BAKING PAPER OR PARCHMENT PAPER

Baking paper is indispensable for baking. Not only does it protect the ingredients from burning or baking too quickly, but also making the cleaning process after baking a piece of cake!

KNOW YOUR MEASUREMENTS

American cooks use standard containers, the 8-ounce cup and a tablespoon that takes exactly 16 level fillings to fill that cup level. Measuring by cup makes it very difficult to give weight equivalents, as the density plays an important role when it comes to weight. The easiest way therefore to deal with cup measurements in recipes is to take the amount by volume rather than by weight. Thus, the equation reads:

1 cup = 240ml = 8 fluid Ounces

½ cup = 120ml = 4 fluid ounces

It is possible to buy a set of American cup measures in major stores around the world.

In the States, butter is sometimes measured in sticks. One stick is the equivalent of 8 tablespoons. One tablespoon of butter is therefore the equivalent to ½ ounce/15 grams.

Liquid Measures

1 Teaspoon= 5 Millilitres

1 Tablespoon = 14 millilitres

2 Tablespoons= 1 Fluid Ounce

Solid Measures

1 Ounce= 28 Grams

16 Ounces= 1 Pound

COOKIE RECIPES

Almond Blueberry Cookies

Total Time Taken: 1 ¼ hours
Yield: 20 Servings
Ingredients:

- ½ cup butter, softened
- 1 teaspoon lemon zest
- 1 egg
- ¼ cup whole milk
- 1 teaspoon almond extract
- 1 ¼ cups all-purpose flour
- 1 cup ground almonds
- ¼ teaspoon salt
- ½ teaspoon baking soda
- ½ cup dried blueberries
- ¼ cup sliced almonds
- 2/3 cup white sugar

Directions:

1. Mix the butter, sugar and lemon zest in a container until fluffy and pale.
2. Put in the egg and milk and mix thoroughly then fold in the flour, ground almonds, baking soda, salt and blueberries.
3. Drop spoonfuls of batter on a baking tray covered with parchment paper and top each cookie with almond slices.
4. Preheat your oven and bake the cookies at 350F for about fifteen minutes or until a golden-brown colour is achieved and fragrant.
5. Serve Chilled or store them in an airtight container for maximum 1 week.

Nutritional Content of One Serving:
Calories: 136 | Fat: 8.0g | Protein: 2.5g | Carbohydrates: 14.6g

Almond Cookies

Total Time Taken: 1 ¼ hours
Yield: 20 Servings
Ingredients:

- ½ cup butter, softened
- 1 teaspoon almond extract
- 2 egg yolks
- 1 ½ cups all-purpose flour
- ½ cup almond flour
- ¼ teaspoon salt
- 1 teaspoon baking powder
- ½ cup sliced almonds
- 2/3 cup white sugar

Directions:

1. Mix the butter, sugar and almond extract in a container until fluffy and pale.
2. Put in the egg yolks and stir thoroughly until blended.
3. Fold in the flours, salt and baking powder.
4. Drop spoonfuls of batter on a baking sheet coated with baking paper.
5. Top each cookie with sliced almonds and preheat your oven and bake at 350F for about fifteen minutes until a golden-brown colour is achieved on the edges.
6. *These cookies taste best chilled.*

Nutritional Content of One Serving:
Calories: 124 | Fat: 6.7g | Protein: 1.9g | Carbohydrates: 14.7g

Amaretti Cookies

Total Time Taken: 1 ¼ hours
Yield: 10 Servings
Ingredients:

- ¼ cup all-purpose flour
- ¼ teaspoon salt 2 egg whites
- ½ cup light brown sugar
- ½ teaspoon baking powder
- 1 teaspoon vanilla extract
- 2 cups almond flour

Directions:

1. Whip the egg whites with salt and vanilla in a container until fluffy.
2. Put in the sugar and continue mixing until shiny and firm.
3. Drop spoonfuls of batter on a baking tray coated with baking paper.
4. Pre-heat the oven and bake at 350F for about twenty minutes or until a golden-brown colour is achieved and crisp.
5. *These cookies taste best chilled.*

Nutritional Content of One Serving:
Calories: 76 | Fat: 2.8g | Protein: 2.2g | Carbohydrates: 10.9g

Amaretti Cookies

Total Time Taken: 1 hour
Yield: 10 Servings
Ingredients:

- 2 cups almond flour
- 1 teaspoon vanilla extract
- ½ teaspoon almond extract
- 2 egg whites
- 2/3 cup light brown sugar

Directions:

1. Mix the egg whites until fluffy.
2. Put in the vanilla and sugar and continue whipping until shiny and firm.

3. Fold in the almond flour then drop spoonfuls of batter on a baking tray coated with baking paper.
4. Preheat your oven and bake the cookies at 350F for about fifteen minutes or until a golden-brown colour is achieved on the edges.
5. *These cookies taste best chilled.*

Nutritional Content of One Serving:
Calories: 74 | Fat: 2.8g | Protein: 1.9g | Carbohydrates: 10.8g

American Chocolate Chunk Cookies

Total Time Taken: 1 ¼ hours
Yield: 20 Servings
Ingredients:

- ½ cup smooth peanut butter
- ½ cup light brown sugar
- 1 egg
- 1 teaspoon vanilla extract
- 1 cup all-purpose flour
- ¼ teaspoon salt
- ½ teaspoon baking powder
- ½ cup peanuts, chopped
- 3 oz. dark chocolate, chopped
- 1/3 cup butter, softened

Directions:

1. Mix the peanut butter, butter and sugar in a container until fluffy and creamy.
2. Put in the egg and vanilla and mix thoroughly.
3. Fold in the flour, salt, baking powder, peanuts and dark chocolate.
4. Drop spoonfuls of batter on a baking tray coated with baking paper.
5. Preheat your oven and bake the cookies at 350F for about fifteen minutes or until a golden-brown colour is achieved on the edges.
6. *These cookies taste best chilled.*

Nutritional Content of One Serving:
Calories: 149 | Fat: 9.7g | Protein: 3.9g | Carbohydrates: 12.8g

Anzac Cookies

Total Time Taken: 1 ¼ hours
Yield: 20 Servings
Ingredients:

- ¼ teaspoon salt
- ½ cup shredded coconut
- ½ teaspoon baking soda
- ¾ cup all-purpose flour
- ¾ cup butter, melted
- 1 cup rolled oats
- 1 teaspoon lemon juice
- 4 tablespoons golden syrup

Directions:

1. Mix the oats, coconut, flour, baking soda and salt in a container.
2. Put in the rest of the ingredients and mix thoroughly.
3. Make small balls of dough and place them in a baking tray coated with baking paper.
4. Flatten the cookies slightly then preheat your oven and bake at 350F for about fifteen minutes or until a golden-brown colour is achieved on the edges.
5. *These cookies taste best chilled.*

Nutritional Content of One Serving:
Calories: 112 | Fat: 7.9g | Protein: 1.2g | Carbohydrates: 9.8g

Apricot Coconut Cookies

Total Time Taken: 1 ½ hours
Yield: 25 Servings
Ingredients:

- ¼ cup light brown sugar
- ¼ teaspoon salt
- ½ cup butter, softened
- ½ cup dark chocolate chips
- ½ cup dried apricots, chopped
- ½ cup rolled oats
- ½ cup white sugar
- ½ teaspoon baking soda
- 1 cup all-purpose flour
- 1 cup shredded coconut
- 1 teaspoon vanilla extract
- 2 eggs

Directions:

1. Mix the flour, coconut, oats, apricots, salt and baking soda in a container.
2. In a separate container, mix the butter and the sugars and vanilla and mix thoroughly.
3. Fold in the flour mixture and the chocolate chips.
4. Drop spoonful of batter on a baking sheet coated with baking paper.
5. Pre-heat the oven and bake at 350F for about fifteen minutes or until a golden-brown colour is achieved on the edges.
6. Let the cookies cool before you serve.

Nutritional Content of One Serving:
Calories: 107 | Fat: 5.9g | Protein: 1.5g | Carbohydrates: 12.8g

Banana Chocolate Chip Cookies

Total Time Taken: 1 ¼ hours
Yield: 20 Servings
Ingredients:

- ¼ teaspoon salt
- ½ cup butter, melted
- ½ cup dark chocolate chips
- ½ cup white sugar

- 1 ½ cups all-purpose flour
- 1 egg
- 1 teaspoon baking powder
- 1 teaspoon vanilla extract
- 2 bananas, mashed

Directions:

1. Combine all the dry ingredients in a container.
2. Put in the rest of the ingredients and mix thoroughly using a spatula.
3. Drop spoonfuls of batter on a baking tray covered with parchment paper.
4. Preheat your oven and bake the cookies at 350F for about fifteen minutes or until a golden-brown colour is achieved on the edges.
5. *These cookies taste best chilled.*

Nutritional Content of One Serving:

Calories: 122 | Fat: 5.8g | Protein: 1.6g | Carbohydrates: 17.0g

Banana Chocolate Cookies

Total Time Taken: 1 ¼ hours

Yield: 20 Servings

Ingredients:

- ¼ cup butter, softened
- ¼ cup cocoa powder
- ¼ cup coconut oil, melted
- ¼ teaspoon baking soda
- ¼ teaspoon salt
- ½ cup walnuts, chopped
- ½ teaspoon baking powder
- 1 ¾ cups all-purpose flour
- 2 bananas, mashed
- 2/3 cup white sugar

Directions:

1. **Mix** the butter, oil and sugar in a container until creamy and fluffy.
2. **Stir in** the bananas then fold in the flour, baking soda, baking powder, salt and cocoa powder.
3. Put in the walnuts then drop spoonfuls of batter on a baking sheet **coated with baking paper**.
4. **Preheat your oven and bake the cookies at** 350F for **fifteen minutes** or **until aromatic**.
5. **These cookies taste best chilled**.

Nutritional Content of One Serving:

Calories: 141 | Fat: 7.2g | Protein: 2.2g | Carbohydrates: 18.7g

Banana Oatmeal Cookies

Total Time Taken: 1 hour

Yield: 10 Servings

Ingredients:

- ¼ teaspoon baking soda
- 1 cup rolled oats
- 1 pinch salt
- 2 tablespoons maple syrup
- 3 ripe bananas, mashed

Directions:

1. Combine all the ingredients in a container.
2. Drop spoonfuls of batter on a baking sheet coated with baking paper.
3. Preheat your oven and bake the cookies at 350F for about ten minutes or until a golden-brown colour is achieved on the edges.
4. *These cookies taste best chilled.*

Nutritional Content of One Serving:

Calories: 73 | Fat: 0.7g | Protein: 1.5g | Carbohydrates: 16.3g

Brown Butter American Cookies

Total Time Taken: 1 ¼ hours

Yield: 20 Servings

Ingredients:

- ¼ teaspoon salt
- ½ cup pecans, chopped
- ½ teaspoon baking soda
- 1 ½ cups all-purpose flour
- 1 cup butter
- 1 cup light brown sugar
- 1 egg
- 1 teaspoon vanilla extract

Directions:

1. Put the butter in a saucepan and melt it then cook it until golden and caramelized. Let cool and then move to a container.
2. Mix the butter and sugar in a fluffy and pale.
3. Put in the egg and vanilla and mix thoroughly then mix in the flour, baking soda, salt and pecans.
4. Drop spoonfuls of batter on a baking tray coated with baking paper.
5. Pre-heat the oven and bake at 350F for about fifteen minutes or until a golden-brown colour is achieved on the edges.
6. *These cookies taste best chilled.*

Nutritional Content of One Serving:

Calories: 152 | Fat: 10.0g | Protein: 1.4g | Carbohydrates: 14.4g

Brown Butter Chocolate Chip Cookies

Total Time Taken: 2 hours

Yield: 20 Servings

Ingredients:

- ¼ teaspoon salt
- ½ cup butter
- ½ teaspoon baking soda
- 1 ½ cups all-purpose flour
- 1 cup dark chocolate chips
- 1 cup light brown sugar
- 1 egg
- 1 egg yolk
- 1 teaspoon baking powder

- 1 teaspoon vanilla extract

Directions:

1. Mix the flour, baking powder, baking soda and salt in a container.
2. Melt the butter in a saucepan until it starts to appear somewhat golden-brown and caramelized. Let cool and then move to a container.
3. Stir in the sugar, egg, egg yolk, vanilla and flour. Stir slowly until mixed using a spatula.
4. Fold in the chocolate chips then drop spoonfuls of dough on a baking sheet coated with baking paper.
5. Freeze the cookies for about half an hour then preheat your oven and bake at 350F for fifteen minutes until a golden-brown colour is achieved. Best served chilled.

Nutritional Content of One Serving:

Calories: 137 | Fat: 6.8g | Protein: 1.8g | Carbohydrates: 18.5g

Brown Butter Chocolate Oatmeal Cookies

Total Time Taken: 1 ¼ hours

Yield: 30 Servings

Ingredients:

- ¼ teaspoon salt
- ½ cup dark chocolate chips
- 1 1/2 cups rolled oats
- 1 cup all-purpose flour
- 1 cup butter
- 1 cup light brown sugar
- 1 egg
- 1 teaspoon baking soda
- 1 teaspoon vanilla extract

Directions:

1. Melt the butter in a saucepan until it becomes mildly golden.
2. Put in the sugar and mix thoroughly then mix in the egg and vanilla.
3. Put in the oats, flour, baking soda and salt then fold in the chocolate chips.
4. Drop spoonfuls of batter on a baking tray coated with baking paper.
5. Preheat your oven and bake the cookies at 350F for about fifteen minutes or until a golden-brown colour is achieved on the edges.
6. *These cookies taste best chilled.*

Nutritional Content of One Serving:

Calories: 115 | Fat: 7.1g | Protein: 1.4g | Carbohydrates: 12.0g

Brown Sugar Chocolate Chip Cookies

Total Time Taken: 1 ½ hours

Yield: 40 Servings

Ingredients:

- ½ cup white sugar
- ½ teaspoon salt
- 1 ½ cups butter, softened
- 1 ½ cups dark chocolate chips
- 1 cup dark brown sugar
- 1 cup light brown sugar
- 1 teaspoon baking soda
- 1 teaspoon vanilla extract
- 2 eggs
- 3 cups all-purpose flour

Directions:

1. Mix the butter and sugars in a container until creamy and fluffy.
2. Put in the eggs and vanilla and mix thoroughly then fold in the remaining ingredients.
3. Drop spoonfuls of batter on a baking tray coated with baking paper.
4. Preheat your oven and bake the cookies at 350F for about fifteen minutes or until a golden-brown colour is achieved on the edges and crisp.
5. *These cookies taste best chilled.*

Nutritional Content of One Serving:

Calories: 157 | Fat: 8.4g | Protein: 1.6g | Carbohydrates: 19.8g

Butter Vanilla Cookies

Total Time Taken: 1 hour

Yield: 30 Servings

Ingredients:

- ¼ cup cornstarch
- ¼ teaspoon salt
- ½ cup powdered sugar
- 1 cup butter, softened
- 1 egg
- 1 tablespoon vanilla extract
- 2 cups all-purpose flour

Directions:

1. Mix the butter and sugar in a container until fluffy and creamy.
2. Put in the egg and vanilla and mix thoroughly.
3. Fold in the flour, cornstarch and salt and mix thoroughly.
4. Drop spoonfuls of batter on a baking sheet coated with baking paper.
5. Pre-heat the oven and bake at 350F for about fifteen minutes or until a golden-brown colour is achieved on the edges.
6. *These cookies taste best chilled.*

Nutritional Content of One Serving:

Calories: 100 | Fat: 6.4g | Protein: 1.1g | Carbohydrates: 9.4g

Cakey Chocolate Chip Cookies

Total Time Taken: 1 hour

Yield: 20 Servings

Ingredients:

- ¼ cup coconut oil, melted

- ¼ cup whole milk
- ¼ teaspoon salt
- ½ cup dark chocolate chips
- ½ cup white sugar
- ½ teaspoon baking powder
- 1 ½ cups all-purpose flour
- 1 egg

Directions:

1. Mix the egg and sugar in a container until volume increases to twice what it was.
2. Put in the coconut oil and milk and mix thoroughly.
3. Stir in the remaining ingredients then drop spoonfuls of batter on a baking tray coated with baking paper.
4. Preheat your oven and bake the cookies at 350F for about ten minutes or until it rises and appears golden.
5. Let cool in the pan before you serve.

Nutritional Content of One Serving:

Calories: 96 | Fat: 3.9g | Protein: 1.6g | Carbohydrates: 14.4g

Candied Ginger Oatmeal Cookies

Total Time Taken: 1 hour

Yield: 30 Servings

Ingredients:

- ¼ cup butter, softened
- ½ cup candied ginger, chopped
- ½ cup canola oil
- ½ teaspoon salt
- 1 cup light brown sugar
- 1 teaspoon baking soda
- 1 teaspoon vanilla extract
- 2 cups all-purpose flour
- 2 cups rolled oats
- 2 eggs

Directions:

1. Mix the butter and sugar in a container until creamy and pale.
2. Put in the eggs and mix thoroughly then mix in the vanilla.
3. Fold in the dry ingredients and ginger then drop spoonfuls of batter on a baking sheet coated with baking paper.
4. Preheat your oven and bake the cookies at 350F for about fifteen minutes or until it is aromatic and appears golden-brown on the edges.
5. *These cookies taste best chilled.*

Nutritional Content of One Serving:

Calories: 121 | Fat: 5.9g | Protein: 2.0g | Carbohydrates: 15.0g

Candy Cane Chocolate Cookies

Total Time Taken: 1 ¼ hours

Yield: 20 Servings

Ingredients:

- ¼ cup cocoa powder
- ¼ cup shredded coconut
- ¼ teaspoon salt
- ½ cup butter, softened
- ½ cup crushed candy cane cookies
- ½ teaspoon baking soda
- 1 cup all-purpose flour
- 1 egg
- 1 teaspoon vanilla extract
- 2 tablespoons canola oil
- 2/3 cup light brown sugar

Directions:

1. Mix the butter, canola oil, sugar and vanilla in a container until fluffy and creamy.
2. Stir in the egg then put in the flour, cocoa powder, coconut, baking soda and salt.
3. Fold in the crushed candy then drop spoonfuls of batter on a baking sheet coated with baking paper.
4. Preheat your oven and bake the cookies at 350F for about fifteen minutes or until aromatic and risen.
5. *These cookies taste best chilled.*

Nutritional Content of One Serving:

Calories: 108 | Fat: 7.0g | Protein: 1.3g | Carbohydrates: 10.8g

Cardamom Chocolate Chip Cookies

Total Time Taken: 1 hour

Yield: 20 Servings

Ingredients:

- ½ cup light brown sugar
- ½ cup white sugar
- ½ teaspoon salt
- 1 cup butter, softened
- 1 cup dark chocolate chips
- 1 teaspoon baking powder
- 1 teaspoon cardamom powder
- 2 ½ cups all-purpose flour
- 2 eggs

Directions:

1. Mix the butter and sugars in a container until creamy and fluffy.
2. Stir in the eggs, one at a time, then put in the flour, salt, baking powder and cardamom powder.
3. Fold in the chocolate chips then drop spoonfuls of batter on a baking sheet coated with baking paper.
4. Pre-heat the oven and bake at 350F for about fifteen minutes.
5. Let the cookies cool in the pan before you serve.

Nutritional Content of One Serving:

Calories: 206 | Fat: 11.4g | Protein: 2.7g | Carbohydrates: 24.7g

Cashew Cranberry Cookies

Total Time Taken: 1 ¼ house
Yield: 30 Servings
Ingredients:

- ¼ teaspoon salt
- ½ cup all-purpose flour
- ½ cup baking soda
- ½ cup coconut oil, melted
- ½ cup light brown sugar
- 1 ½ cups ground cashew nuts
- 1 cup dried cranberries
- 1 teaspoon vanilla extract
- 2 eggs
- 2 tablespoons golden syrup

Directions:

1. Mix the cashew nuts, flour, salt and baking soda in a container.
2. In a separate container, combine the coconut oil, eggs, vanilla, sugar and syrup until creamy.
3. Put in the flour mixture then fold in the cranberries.
4. Drop spoonfuls of batter on a baking sheet coated with baking paper.
5. Preheat your oven and bake the cookies at 350F for about fifteen minutes or until a golden-brown colour is achieved on the edges.
6. *These cookies taste best chilled.*

Nutritional Content of One Serving:
Calories: 106 | Fat: 7.7g | Protein: 2.0g | Carbohydrates: 7.6g

Chewy Coconut Cookies

Total Time Taken: 1 hour
Yield: 20 Servings
Ingredients:

- ¼ cup coconut oil, melted
- ¼ cup cornstarch
- ¼ teaspoon salt
- ½ teaspoon baking soda
- ½ teaspoon coconut extract
- 1 ¼ cups all-purpose flour
- 1 cup shredded coconut
- 1 cup white sugar
- 1 egg
- 1 teaspoon vanilla extract

Directions:

1. Mix the egg and sugar in a container until volume increases to twice what it was. Stir in the coconut oil then put in the coconut oil, vanilla and coconut extract.
2. Fold in the flour, cornstarch, baking soda, salt and coconut.
3. Drop spoonfuls of batter on a baking sheet pan coated with baking paper.
4. Preheat your oven and bake the cookies at 350F for about fifteen minutes or until a golden-brown colour is achieved on the edges.
5. *These cookies taste best chilled.*

Nutritional Content of One Serving:
Calories: 114 | Fat: 4.4g | Protein: 1.2g | Carbohydrates: 18.1g

Chewy Sugar Cookies

Total Time Taken: 1 ¼ hours
Yield: 40 Servings
Ingredients:

- ½ teaspoon salt
- 1 cup butter, softened
- 1 teaspoon baking soda
- 1 teaspoon vanilla extract
- 2 ½ cups all-purpose flour
- 2 cups white sugar
- 2 eggs

Directions:

1. Mix the butter with sugar until creamy and pale. Put in the eggs, one at a time, then mix in the vanilla.
2. Fold in the flour, baking soda and salt then shape the dough into small balls.
3. Put the balls on a baking tray coated with baking paper and flatten them slightly.
4. Preheat your oven and bake the cookies at 350F for about fifteen minutes or until mildly golden brown.
5. *These cookies taste best chilled.*

Nutritional Content of One Serving:
Calories: 110 | Fat: 4.9g | Protein: 1.1g | Carbohydrates: 16.0g

Chili Chocolate Cookies

Total Time Taken: 1 ¼ hours
Yield: 30 Servings
Ingredients:

- ¼ cup dark brown sugar
- ½ cup cocoa powder
- ½ cup white sugar
- ½ teaspoon salt
- 1 cup butter, softened
- 1 cup dark chocolate chips
- 1 teaspoon baking powder
- 1 teaspoon chili powder
- 1 teaspoon vanilla extract
- 2 cups all-purpose flour
- 2 eggs

Directions:

1. Mix the butter and sugars in a container until creamy and fluffy.
2. Put in the vanilla and eggs and mix thoroughly.

3. Fold in the flour, cocoa powder, salt, chili powder and baking powder then put in the chocolate chips.
4. Drop spoonfuls of batter on a baking sheet coated with baking paper.
5. Preheat your oven and bake the cookies at 350F for about fifteen minutes or until risen and fragrant.
6. *These cookies taste best chilled.*

Nutritional Content of One Serving:
Calories: 129 | Fat: 7.8g | Protein: 1.8g | Carbohydrates: 14.5g

Chocolate Buttercream Cookies

Total Time Taken: 1 ½ hours
Yield: 20 Servings
Ingredients:
Cookies:

- ½ cup butter, softened
- ½ cup cocoa powder
- ½ cup coconut oil
- ½ cup powdered sugar
- ½ teaspoon baking powder
- ½ teaspoon salt
- 1 egg
- 2 cups all-purpose flour
- 2 tablespoons whole milk

Filling:

- ½ cup butter, softened
- 1 cup powdered sugar

Directions:
1. For the cookies, combine the flour, cocoa powder, salt and baking powder in a container.
2. In a separate container, combine the coconut oil, butter and sugar in a container until creamy and fluffy.
3. Put in the egg and mix thoroughly, then mix in the flour and the milk.
4. Cover the dough with plastic wrap and store in the refrigerator for about half an hour.
5. Transfer the dough to a floured working surface and roll into a slim sheet.
6. Cut small round cookies and place them on a baking sheet.
7. Pre-heat the oven and bake at 350F for about fifteen minutes.
8. Let the cookies cool to room temperature.
9. For the filling, combine the butter with sugar until fluffy and creamy.
10. Fill the cookies, two by two with the buttercream.
11. Serve fresh or store in an airtight container.

Nutritional Content of One Serving:
Calories: 218 | Fat: 15.4g | Protein: 2.1g | Carbohydrates: 19.8g

Chocolate Chip Pecan Cookies

Total Time Taken: 1 ¼ hours
Yield: 20 Servings
Ingredients:

- ¼ teaspoon salt
- ½ cup butter, softened
- ½ cup chocolate chips
- ½ cup powdered sugar
- ½ teaspoon baking soda
- 1 cup all-purpose flour
- 1 cup ground pecans
- 1 egg
- 2 tablespoon honey

Directions:
1. Mix the butter, sugar and honey in a container until creamy and pale.
2. Put in the egg and mix thoroughly then put in the flour, pecans, baking soda and salt.
3. Fold in the chocolate chips then drop spoonfuls of batter on a baking sheet coated with baking paper.
4. Pre-heat the oven and bake at 350F for about fifteen minutes or until a golden-brown colour is achieved and fragrant.
5. *These cookies taste best chilled.*

Nutritional Content of One Serving:
Calories: 112 | Fat: 6.6g | Protein: 1.4g | Carbohydrates: 12.1g

Chocolate Chunk Cookies

Total Time Taken: 1 ¼ hours
Yield: 20 Servings
Ingredients:

- ¼ teaspoon salt
- ½ cup butter, softened
- 1 ½ cups all-purpose flour
- 1 egg
- 1 teaspoon baking powder
- 2 tablespoons honey
- 2/3 cup light brown sugar
- 4 oz. dark chocolate, chopped

Directions:
1. Mix the butter, honey and sugar in a container until fluffy and pale.
2. Put in the egg and mix thoroughly then mix in the flour, baking powder and salt.
3. Fold in the chocolate then drop spoonfuls of dough on a baking sheet coated with baking paper.
4. Preheat your oven and bake the cookies at 350F for fifteen minutes or until a golden-brown colour is achieved on the edges.
5. *These cookies taste best chilled.*

Nutritional Content of One Serving:
Calories: 133 | Fat: 6.6g | Protein: 1.8g | Carbohydrates: 17.1g

Chocolate Crinkles

Total Time Taken: 2 hours
Yield: 40 Servings
Ingredients:

- ½ cup cocoa powder
- ½ cup coconut oil, melted
- ½ teaspoon salt
- 1 ½ teaspoons baking powder
- 1 teaspoon vanilla extract
- 2 cups all-purpose flour
- 2 cups powdered sugar
- 2 cups white sugar
- 4 eggs
- 4 oz. dark chocolate, melted

Directions:

1. Mix the coconut oil and melted chocolate in a container.
2. Put in the sugar and eggs and mix thoroughly then mix in the vanilla.
3. Fold in the flour, baking powder, cocoa and salt then cover the dough using plastic wrap.
4. Place in your refrigerator for an hour then form small balls of dough and roll them through powdered sugar.
5. Put the cookies on a baking tray coated with baking paper and preheat your oven and bake at 350F for about ten minutes.
6. *These cookies taste best chilled.*

Nutritional Content of One Serving:
Calories: 131 | Fat: 4.2g | Protein: 1.6g | Carbohydrates: 23.1g

Chocolate Dipped Sugar Cookies

Total Time Taken: 1 ¼ hours
Yield: 30 Servings
Ingredients:

- ¼ teaspoon salt
- 1 cup butter, softened
- 1 cup dark chocolate, melted
- 1 cup powdered sugar
- 1 teaspoon baking powder
- 1 teaspoon vanilla extract
- 2 egg yolks
- 3 cups all-purpose flour

Directions:

1. Mix the butter and sugar in a container until pale and fluffy.
2. Stir in the egg yolks and vanilla and mix thoroughly.
3. Fold in the flour, baking powder and salt then wrap the dough in plastic wrap and store in the refrigerator for about half an hour.
4. Transfer the dough to a floured working surface and roll into a slim sheet.
5. Cut cookies using a cookie cutter of your choices and arrange them on a baking sheet coated with baking paper.
6. Pre-heat the oven and bake at 350F for about thirteen minutes or until mildly golden-brown on the edges.
7. When finished, allow the cookies to cool then immerse them in melted chocolate.
8. *These cookies taste best chilled.*

Nutritional Content of One Serving:
Calories: 149 | Fat: 8.2g | Protein: 2.0g | Carbohydrates: 17.0g

Chocolate Drizzled Lavender Cookies

Total Time Taken: 1 ½ hours
Yield: 20 Servings
Ingredients:

- ¼ cup cornstarch
- ¼ teaspoon baking soda
- ¼ teaspoon salt
- ½ cup butter, softened
- ½ cup powdered sugar
- ½ cup white chocolate chips, melted
- 1 ½ cups all-purpose flour
- 1 egg
- 1 egg yolk
- 1 teaspoon lavender buds
- 2 tablespoons whole milk

Directions:

1. Mix the butter with sugar in a container until fluffy and pale.
2. Stir in the egg and egg yolk and mix thoroughly.
3. Put in the milk and mix then fold in the remaining ingredients. Mix the dough then move it to a floured working surface and roll it into a slim sheet.
4. Cut into small cookies using a cookie cutter of your choices.
5. Position the cookies on a baking sheet coated with baking paper.
6. Pre-heat the oven and bake at 350F for about fifteen minutes or until a golden-brown colour is achieved on the edges.
7. When finished, let cool in the pan then sprinkle the cookies with melted chocolate.
8. **Best served chilled.**

Nutritional Content of One Serving:
Calories: 122 | Fat: 6.6g | Protein: 1.7g | Carbohydrates: 14.2g

Chocolate Hazelnut Cookies

Total Time Taken: 1 ½ hours
Yield: 30 Servings
Ingredients:

- ¼ cup cocoa powder
- ¼ teaspoon salt

- ½ cup cream cheese, softened
- ½ cup ground hazelnuts
- 1 ½ cups all-purpose flour
- 1 cup butter, softened
- 1 egg yolk

Directions:

1. Mix the butter, cream cheese and egg yolk in a container until creamy.
2. Put in the salt, flour, cocoa powder and hazelnuts and mix using a spatula.
3. Wrap the plastic wrap and store in the refrigerator for about half an hour.
4. Transfer the dough to a floured working surface and roll it into a slim sheet.
5. Cut into small cookies with a cookie cutter of your choices.
6. Put the cookies in a baking sheet coated with baking paper and preheat your oven and bake at 350F for about ten minutes or until a golden-brown colour is achieved on the edges.
7. *These cookies taste best chilled.*

Nutritional Content of One Serving:

Calories: 102 | Fat: 8.6g | Protein: 1.4g | Carbohydrates: 5.5g

Chocolate Nutella Cookies

Total Time Taken: 1 ¼ hours
Yield: 30 Servings
Ingredients:

- ¼ cup cocoa powder
- ¼ cup white sugar
- ½ teaspoon baking soda
- ½ teaspoon salt
- ¾ cup light brown sugar
- 1 cup butter, softened
- 1 cup dark chocolate chips
- 1 cup Nutella
- 1 teaspoon vanilla extract
- 2 cups all-purpose flour
- 2 eggs

Directions:

1. Mix the butter and sugars in a container until creamy and fluffy.
2. Put in the Nutella, vanilla and eggs and mix thoroughly.
3. Fold in the remaining ingredients then drop spoonfuls of batter on a baking tray covered with parchment paper.
4. Preheat your oven and bake the cookies at 350F for about fifteen minutes or until a golden-brown colour is achieved.
5. *Serve the cookie chilled.*

Nutritional Content of One Serving:

Calories: 136 | Fat: 8.0g | Protein: 1.8g | Carbohydrates: 15.5g

Chocolate Orange Shortbread Cookies

Total Time Taken: 1 hour
Yield: 20 Servings
Ingredients:

- ¼ cup cocoa powder
- ¼ teaspoon salt
- ½ cup almond flour
- ½ cup butter, softened
- ½ cup white sugar
- ½ teaspoon baking soda
- 1 ½ cups all-purpose flour
- 1 egg
- 1 tablespoon orange zest
- 1 teaspoon vanilla extract

Directions:

1. Mix the butter, cocoa powder and sugar in a container until fluffy and pale.
2. Put in the egg, vanilla and orange zest and mix thoroughly.
3. Fold in the flour, almond flour, salt and baking soda then transfer the dough on a floured working surface.
4. Roll the dough into a slim sheet then cut small cookies using a cookie cutter of your choice.
5. Preheat your oven and bake the cookies at 350F for about fifteen minutes or until a golden-brown colour is achieved and fragrant.
6. *These cookies taste best chilled.*

Nutritional Content of One Serving:

Calories: 104 | Fat: 5.4g | Protein: 1.6g | Carbohydrates: 13.0g

Chocolate Pecan Cookies

Total Time Taken: 1 hour
Yield: 10 Servings
Ingredients:

- ¼ teaspoon salt
- ½ cup dark chocolate chips
- 1 cup ground pecans
- 1 teaspoon vanilla extract
- 2 egg whites
- 2/3 cup white sugar

Directions:

1. Whip the egg whites and salt in a container until fluffy and airy.
2. Put in the sugar, progressively, and stir until shiny.
3. Fold in the pecans and chocolate chips then drop spoonfuls of batter on a baking sheet coated with baking paper.
4. Preheat your oven and bake the cookies at 350F for about fifteen minutes or until a golden-brown colour is achieved.
5. *These cookies taste best chilled.*

Nutritional Content of One Serving:

Calories: 92 | Fat: 2.6g | Protein: 1.3g | Carbohydrates: 17.6g

Chocolate Sandwich Cookies With Passionfruit Ganache

Total Time Taken: 2 hours
Yield: 30 Servings
Ingredients:
Cookies:
- ½ cup cocoa powder
- ½ teaspoon salt
- 1 cup white sugar
- 1 egg
- 1 teaspoon baking powder
- 1 teaspoon vanilla extract
- 2 cups all-purpose flour
- 2/3 cup butter, softened

Passionfruit Ganache:
- ¼ cup passionfruit juice
- ½ cup heavy cream
- 1 cup white chocolate chips
- 2 tablespoons butter

Directions:
1. For the cookies, combine the flour, cocoa powder, baking powder and salt in a container.
1. In a separate container, combine the butter and sugar until fluffy and pale.
2. Stir in the egg and vanilla and mix thoroughly then fold in the flour.
3. Transfer the dough to a floured working surface and roll it into a slim sheet.
4. Cut 40 small cookies using a round cookie cutter and arrange them on a baking sheet coated with baking paper.
5. For the ganache, bring the cream to a boil. Stir in the chocolate and stir until it melts completely. Put in the passionfruit juice and butter and mix thoroughly. Let cool in your refrigerator.
6. Fill the cookies with chilled ganache.

Nutritional Content of One Serving:
Calories: 143 | Fat: 7.8g | Protein: 1.7g | Carbohydrates: 17.6g

Chocolate Star Anise Cookies

Total Time Taken: 1 ¼ hours
Yield: 20 Servings
Ingredients:
- ½ cup butter, softened
- ½ cup cocoa powder
- ½ cup pecans, chopped
- ½ teaspoon baking soda
- ½ teaspoon salt
- ¾ cup white sugar
- 1 ½ cups all-purpose flour
- 1 egg
- 1 teaspoon ground star anise
- 2 tablespoons coconut oil

Directions:
1. Mix the butter and coconut oil in a container. Put in the sugar and stir until fluffy.
2. Stir in the egg and stir thoroughly until blended.
3. Fold in the remaining ingredients and mix using a spatula.
4. Drop spoonfuls of batter on baking trays covered with parchment paper.
5. Pre-heat the oven and bake at 350F for about fifteen minutes or until risen and fragrant.
6. *These cookies taste best chilled.*

Nutritional Content of One Serving:
Calories: 129 | Fat: 7.1g | Protein: 1.8g | Carbohydrates: 16.1g

Chunky Peanut Butter Cookies

Total Time Taken: 1 ¼ hours
Yield: 30 Servings
Ingredients:
- ¼ teaspoon salt
- ½ cup butter, softened
- 1 cup light brown sugar
- 1 cup peanut butter, softened
- 1 cup peanuts, chopped
- 1 egg
- 1 teaspoon baking powder
- 2 cups all-purpose flour

Directions:
1. Mix the butter and peanut butter in a container until creamy. Put in the sugar and mix for five minutes until fluffy.
2. Put in the egg and mix thoroughly then fold in the remaining ingredients.
3. Drop spoonfuls of batter on a baking tray coated with baking paper.
4. Preheat your oven and bake the cookies at 350F for about fifteen minutes or until a golden-brown colour is achieved on the edges.
5. Allow the cookies cool down before you serve.

Nutritional Content of One Serving:
Calories: 156 | Fat: 10.0g | Protein: 4.5g | Carbohydrates: 13.7g

Cinnamon Oatmeal Cookies

Total Time Taken: 1 ¼ hours
Yield: 30 Servings
Ingredients:
- ¼ cup golden syrup
- 1 egg
- 2 cups rolled oats
- 1 teaspoon cinnamon powder
- ¼ teaspoon salt
- ½ teaspoon baking soda

- 2/3 cup butter
- 2/3 cup light brown sugar
- 2/3 cup all-purpose flour

Directions:

1. Mix the butter, sugar and syrup in a container until fluffy and creamy.
2. Put in the egg and mix thoroughly then fold in the remaining ingredients.
3. Drop spoonfuls of batter on a baking sheet coated with baking paper.
4. Preheat your oven and bake the cookies at 350F for about fifteen minutes or until a golden-brown colour is achieved on the edges.
5. Let the cookies cool down before you serve.

Nutritional Content of One Serving:

Calories: 89 | Fat: 4.6g | Protein: 1.2g | Carbohydrates: 11.1g

Cinnamon Snap Cookies

Total Time Taken: 1 ¼ hours

Yield: 30 Servings

Ingredients:

- ¼ cup cocoa powder
- ½ teaspoon ground cloves
- ½ teaspoon ground ginger
- ½ teaspoon salt
- 1 cup butter, softened
- 1 egg
- 1 teaspoon baking soda
- 1 teaspoon cinnamon powder
- 1 teaspoon vanilla extract
- 2 cups all-purpose flour
- 2 tablespoons golden syrup
- 2/3 cup white sugar

Directions:

1. Mix the butter, sugar, vanilla and golden syrup in a container until pale and creamy.
2. Put in the egg and mix thoroughly then put in the flour mixture.
3. Make small balls of dough and place the cookies on a baking sheet coated with baking paper.
4. Preheat your oven and bake the cookies at 350F for about fifteen minutes until it is aromatic and appears golden brown.
5. *These cookies taste best chilled.*

Nutritional Content of One Serving:

Calories: 109 | Fat: 6.5g | Protein: 1.2g | Carbohydrates: 12.3g

Cinnamon Sugar Cookies

Total Time Taken: 1 ½ hours

Yield: 25 Servings

Ingredients:

- ¼ teaspoon salt
- ½ cup coconut oil, melted
- ½ cup light brown sugar
- 1 cup white sugar
- 1 teaspoon baking powder
- 1 teaspoon cinnamon powder
- 1 teaspoon vanilla extract
- 2 cups all-purpose flour
- 2 eggs

Directions:

1. Mix the brown sugar and cinnamon in a container and set aside for later.
2. Combine the eggs and sugar in a separate container and stir until volume increases to twice what it was.
3. Put in the coconut oil and vanilla and mix thoroughly.
4. Put in the flour, salt and baking powder and mix using a spatula.
5. Make small balls of dough and roll them through cinnamon sugar.
6. Preheat your oven and bake the cookies at 350F for about fifteen minutes or until a golden-brown colour is achieved and fragrant.
7. *These cookies taste best chilled.*

Nutritional Content of One Serving:

Calories: 121 | Fat: 4.8g | Protein: 1.5g | Carbohydrates: 18.6g

Clove Sugar Cookies

Total Time Taken: 1 ¼ hours

Yield: 30 Servings

Ingredients:

- ¼ teaspoon salt
- ½ cup powdered sugar
- ½ teaspoon baking powder
- 1 cup butter, softened
- 1 cup ground hazelnuts
- 1 egg yolk
- 1 teaspoon ground whole cloves
- 1 teaspoon vanilla extract
- 2 cups all-purpose flour

Directions:

1. Mix the butter and sugar in a container until pale and fluffy.
2. Put in the vanilla and egg yolk and mix thoroughly.
3. Fold in the flour, hazelnuts, cloves, salt and baking powder.
4. Transfer the dough to a floured working surface then roll the dough into a slim sheet.
5. Cut into small cookies with a cookie cutter and place them on a baking tray coated with baking paper.
6. Preheat your oven and bake the cookies at 350F for about fifteen minutes or until a golden-brown colour is achieved and fragrant.
7. *These cookies taste best chilled.*

Nutritional Content of One Serving:

Calories: 115 | Fat: 7.9g | Protein: 1.5g | Carbohydrates: 9.7g

Coconut Butter Cookies

Total Time Taken: 1 ¼ hours
Yield: 20 Servings
Ingredients:

- ¼ teaspoon salt
- ½ cup coconut butter, softened
- 1 cup shredded coconut
- 1 egg
- 1 teaspoon baking powder
- 1 teaspoon coconut extract
- 2 cups all-purpose flour
- 2 tablespoons coconut oil
- 2/3 cup white sugar

Directions:

1. Mix the coconut butter, coconut oil and sugar in a container until pale and creamy.
2. Put in the egg and coconut extract and mix thoroughly.
3. Stir in the flour, coconut, baking powder and salt then form small balls of dough.
4. Put the balls on baking trays coated with baking paper and preheat your oven and bake at 350F for about fifteen minutes or until a golden-brown colour is achieved,
5. When finished, transfer the cookies in a container and dust them with powdered sugar.
6. *These cookies taste best chilled.*

Nutritional Content of One Serving:
Calories: 100 | Fat: 3.0g | Protein: 1.7g | Carbohydrates: 17.0g

Coconut Florentine Cookies

Total Time Taken: 1 ¼ hours
Yield: 25 Servings
Ingredients:

- ¼ cup honey
- ¼ teaspoon salt
- ½ cup light brown sugar
- 1 ½ cups sliced almonds
- 1 cup butter, softened
- 1 cup shredded coconut
- 4 tablespoons all-purpose flour

Directions:

1. Mix the butter, sugar and honey in a heatproof container over a hot water bath until smooth and melted.
2. Turn off the heat and put in the coconut, almonds, salt and flour.
3. Drop spoonfuls of batter on a baking tray coated with baking paper.
4. Spread the mixture slightly then preheat your oven and bake the cookies at 350F for about fifteen minutes or until a golden-brown colour is achieved and crisp.
5. Let the cookies cool down before you serve.

Nutritional Content of One Serving:
Calories: 135 | Fat: 11.3g | Protein: 1.5g | Carbohydrates: 8.3g

Coconut Lime Butter Cookies

Total Time Taken: 1 ¼ hours
Yield: 30 Servings
Ingredients:

- ½ teaspoon baking powder
- ½ teaspoon salt
- 1 cup butter, softened
- 1 cup shredded coconut
- 1 cup white sugar
- 1 lime, zested and juiced
- 1 teaspoon coconut extract
- 2 cups all-purpose flour
- 2 egg yolks

Directions:

1. Mix the butter and sugar in a container until creamy and pale.
2. Put in the egg yolks, lime zest and lime juice, as well as the coconut extract.
3. Stir in the flour, salt, coconut and baking powder then transfer the dough on a floured working surface.
4. Roll the dough into a slim sheet then cut small cookies using a cookie cutter of your choice.
5. Put the cookies on a baking tray covered with parchment paper.
6. Preheat your oven and bake the cookies at 350F for about fifteen minutes or until a golden-brown colour is achieved on the edges.
7. *These cookies taste best chilled.*

Nutritional Content of One Serving:
Calories: 124 | Fat: 7.4g | Protein: 1.2g | Carbohydrates: 13.8g

Coconut Macaroons

Total Time Taken: 1 ½ hours
Yield: 20 Servings
Ingredients:

- ¼ teaspoon salt
- ½ cup all-purpose flour
- 1 can sweetened condensed milk
- 1 teaspoon vanilla extract
- 4 cups shredded coconut

Directions:

1. Mix the coconut, salt and flour in a container.
2. Put in the milk and vanilla and mix thoroughly.
3. Drop spoonfuls of mixture on baking trays coated with baking paper.

4. Preheat your oven and bake the cookies at 350F for fifteen minutes or until crisp and golden brown.
5. *These cookies taste best chilled.*

Nutritional Content of One Serving:
Calories: 118 | Fat: 6.7g | Protein: 2.1g | Carbohydrates: 13.2g

Coconut Shortbread Cookies

Total Time Taken: 2 hours
Yield: 20 Servings
Ingredients:

- ¼ teaspoon baking powder
- ¼ teaspoon salt
- ½ cup powdered sugar
- 1 cup butter, softened
- 1 cup shredded coconut
- 1 egg
- 1 teaspoon coconut extract
- 2 cups all-purpose flour

Directions:

1. Mix the butter, sugar and coconut extract in a container.
2. Stir in the egg and mix thoroughly then put in the flour, salt, coconut and baking powder.
3. Wrap the dough in a plastic wrap and store in the refrigerator for about half an hour.
4. Transfer the dough to a working surface and roll it into a slim sheet.
5. Cut the dough into small cookies with a cookie cutter of your choice.
6. Put the cookies in a baking tray coated with baking paper.
7. Pre-heat the oven and bake at 350F for about fifteen minutes or until a golden-brown colour is achieved on the edges.
8. *Best served chilled.*

Nutritional Content of One Serving:
Calories: 157 | Fat: 10.9g | Protein: 1.8g | Carbohydrates: 13.2g

Coffee Gingersnap Cookies

Total Time Taken: 1 ¼ hours
Yield: 20 Servings
Ingredients:

- ¼ cup coconut oil
- ¼ teaspoon salt
- ½ cup butter, softened
- ½ teaspoon ground cardamom
- 1 cup light brown sugar
- 1 egg
- 1 teaspoon baking soda
- 1 teaspoon cinnamon powder
- 1 teaspoon ground ginger
- 1 teaspoon vanilla extract
- 2 cups all-purpose flour
- 2 teaspoons instant coffee

Directions:

1. Mix the butter, coconut oil and brown sugar in a container until fluffy and creamy.
2. Put in the egg and vanilla and mix thoroughly.
3. Fold in the remaining ingredients then drop spoonfuls of batter on a baking sheet coated with baking paper.
4. Pre-heat the oven and bake at 350F for fifteen minutes or until aromatic and crunchy.
5. *These cookies taste best chilled.*

Nutritional Content of One Serving:
Calories: 142 | Fat: 7.7g | Protein: 1.7g | Carbohydrates: 16.8g

Coffee Shortbread Cookies

Total Time Taken: 1 hour
Yield: 20 Servings
Ingredients:

- ½ cup butter, softened
- ½ cup powdered sugar
- ½ teaspoon baking powder
- ½ teaspoon salt
- 1 egg
- 1 teaspoon vanilla extract
- 2 cups all-purpose flour
- 2 teaspoons instant coffee

Directions:

1. Mix the butter, sugar and vanilla and stir until smooth and fluffy.
2. Put in the egg and mix thoroughly then fold in the flour, salt, baking powder and coffee.
3. Put the dough on a floured working surface and roll it into a slim sheet.
4. Cut into small cookies using a cookie cutter of your choices and position the cookies on a baking sheet coated with baking paper.
5. Preheat your oven and bake the cookies at 350F for about fifteen minutes or until it is aromatic and appears golden-brown on the edges.
6. Serve Chilled or store them in an airtight container.

Nutritional Content of One Serving:
Calories: 102 | Fat: 5.0g | Protein: 1.6g | Carbohydrates: 12.6g

Colorful Chocolate Cookies

Total Time Taken: 1 ¼ hors
Yield: 30 Servings
Ingredients:

- ½ cup cocoa powder
- ½ cup crushed candy cane cookies
- ½ cup M&M candies
- ½ teaspoon salt
- 1 cup butter, softened

- 1 cup light brown sugar
- 1 egg
- 1 teaspoon baking powder
- 1 teaspoon vanilla extract
- 2 cups all-purpose flour

Directions:

1. Mix the butter, sugar and vanilla and stir thoroughly until fluffy and pale.
2. Stir in the egg and mix thoroughly then put in the remaining ingredients.
3. Drop spoonfuls of batter on a baking tray coated with baking paper.
4. Pre-heat the oven and bake at 350F for about fifteen minutes.
5. Let the cookies cool in the pan before you serve.

Nutritional Content of One Serving:

Calories: 129 | Fat: 7.4g | Protein: 1.5g | Carbohydrates: 14.8g

Confetti Cookies

Total Time Taken: 1 ¼ hours
Yield: 20 Servings
Ingredients:

- 1 teaspoon vanilla extract
- 1 egg
- 2 cups all-purpose flour
- 1 teaspoon baking powder
- ¼ teaspoon salt
- ½ cup colourful sprinkles
- 2/3 cup butter, softened
- 2/3 cup white sugar

Directions:

1. Mix the butter with sugar and vanilla in a container until creamy and fluffy.
2. Stir in the egg and mix thoroughly then fold in the remaining ingredients.
3. Drop in the sprinkles and mix using a spatula.
4. Drop spoonfuls of batter on a baking sheet coated with baking paper.
5. Pre-heat the oven and bake at 350F for about fifteen minutes or until a golden-brown colour is achieved on the edges.
6. *These cookies taste best chilled.*

Nutritional Content of One Serving:

Calories: 136 | Fat: 6.7g | Protein: 1.7g | Carbohydrates: 17.5g

Cornflake Chocolate Chip Cookies

Total Time Taken: 1 hour
Yield: 20 Servings
Ingredients:

- ½ cup butter, softened
- ½ cup dark chocolate chips
- ½ teaspoon baking soda
- ¾ cup white sugar
- 1 ¼ cup all-purpose flour
- 1 cup cornflakes
- 1 egg
- 1 teaspoon vanilla extract
- 2/4 teaspoon salt

Directions:

1. Mix the butter, sugar and vanilla in a container until creamy and pale.
2. Put in the egg then mix in the flour, baking soda and salt.
3. Fold in the cornflakes and chocolate chips.
4. Drop spoonfuls of batter on a baking sheet coated with baking paper.
5. Preheat your oven and bake the cookies at 350F for about fifteen minutes or until a golden-brown colour is achieved on the edges.
6. *These cookies taste best chilled.*

Nutritional Content of One Serving:

Calories: 120 | Fat: 5.7g | Protein: 1.4g | Carbohydrates: 16.7g

Cracked Sugar Cookies

Total Time Taken: 1 ¼ hours
Yield: 30 Servings
Ingredients:

- ½ teaspoon salt
- 1 cup butter, softened
- 1 cup powdered sugar
- 1 cup white sugar
- 1 teaspoon baking soda
- 1 teaspoon vanilla extract
- 2 ½ cups all-purpose flour
- 3 egg yolks

Directions:

1. Mix the butter and sugar in a container until creamy and fluffy.
2. Put in the egg yolks and mix thoroughly then mix in the vanilla.
3. Fold in the flour, baking soda and salt then form small balls of dough and roll them through powdered sugar.
4. Put the balls on a baking tray coated with baking paper.
5. Pre-heat the oven and bake at 350F for about fifteen minutes or until mildly golden brown.
6. These cookies taste best chilled, handling them with care.

Nutritional Content of One Serving:

Calories: 139 | Fat: 6.7g | Protein: 1.4g | Carbohydrates: 18.7g

Cranberry Biscotti

Total Time Taken: 1 ½ hours
Yield: 20 Servings
Ingredients:

- ¼ teaspoon salt
- ½ cup butter, softened
- ½ cup white sugar
- ½ teaspoon baking soda
- 1 cup dried cranberries
- 1 egg
- 1 tablespoon lemon zest
- 2 cups all-purpose flour

Directions:

1. Mix the butter and sugar in a container until creamy and fluffy.
2. Put in the egg and lemon zest and mix thoroughly.
3. Stir in the flour, baking soda and salt then put in the cranberries.
4. Put the dough on a baking tray coated with baking paper. Shape the dough into a log and bake it in the preheated oven at 350F for fifteen minutes.
5. Remove the tray from the oven and allow it to cool down for about ten minutes. Cut the log into 1cm wide slices and place them back on the tray with the cut facing up.
6. Carry on baking for fifteen minutes or until a golden-brown colour is achieved and crisp.
7. Let cool before you serve or storing.

Nutritional Content of One Serving:

Calories: 111 | Fat: 5.0g | Protein: 1.6g | Carbohydrates: 15.1g

Custard Powder Cookies

Total Time Taken: 1 ¼ hours
Yield: 20 Servings
Ingredients:

- ¼ cup whole milk
- ¼ teaspoon salt
- ½ cup butter, softened
- ½ cup vanilla custard powder
- ½ cup white sugar
- 1 ½ cups all-purpose flour
- 1 teaspoon baking powder
- 1 teaspoon vanilla extract

Directions:

1. Mix the butter and sugar in a container until creamy and fluffy.
2. Stir in the milk and vanilla then fold in the remaining ingredients.
3. Drop spoonfuls of batter on a baking sheet coated with baking paper.
4. Preheat your oven and bake the cookies at 350F for about fifteen minutes or until a golden-brown colour is achieved on the edges.
5. *These cookies taste best chilled.*

Nutritional Content of One Serving:

Calories: 115 | Fat: 4.8g | Protein: 1.1g | Carbohydrates: 17.3g

Date Pecan Ginger Cookies

Total Time Taken: 1 ½ hours
Yield: 30 Servings
Ingredients:

- ¼ teaspoon salt
- ½ cup olive oil
- ½ cup whole wheat flour
- 1 cup all-purpose flour
- 1 cup dates, pitted and chopped
- 1 cup light brown sugar
- 1 cup pecans, chopped
- 1 egg
- 1 teaspoon baking powder
- 1 teaspoon grated ginger
- 1 teaspoon vanilla extract

Directions:

1. Mix the oil and sugar in a container until fluffy and pale.
2. Put in the vanilla and ginger and mix thoroughly then fold in the flours, baking powder and salt.
3. Stir in the dates and pecans then drop spoonfuls of batter on a baking sheet coated with baking paper.
4. Preheat your oven and bake the cookies at 350F for fifteen minutes or until a golden-brown colour is achieved on the edges.
5. *These cookies taste best chilled.*

Nutritional Content of One Serving:

Calories: 93 | Fat: 3.9g | Protein: 1.0g | Carbohydrates: 14.2g

Double Chocolate Cookies

Total Time Taken: 1 ½ hours
Yield: 30 Servings
Ingredients:

- ¼ teaspoon salt
- ½ cup cocoa powder
- ½ cup mini chocolate chips
- ½ teaspoon baking powder
- 1 ½ cups all-purpose flour
- 1 cup white sugar
- 1 egg
- 1 teaspoon vanilla extract
- 2/3 cup butter, softened

Directions:

1. Mix the butter and sugar until fluffy and creamy.
2. Put in the egg and vanilla and mix thoroughly then fold in the remaining ingredients and mix thoroughly.
3. Cover the dough with plastic wrap and store in the refrigerator for about half an hour.
4. Transfer the dough to a floured working surface and roll it into a slim sheet.

5. Cut into small cookies using a cookie cutter of your choices and place them on a baking pan coated with baking paper.
6. Pre-heat the oven and bake at 350F for about fifteen minutes.
7. *These cookies taste best chilled.*

Nutritional Content of One Serving:
Calories: 93 | Fat: 4.6g | Protein: 1.2g | Carbohydrates: 12.8g

Double Chocolate Espresso Cookies

Total Time Taken: 1 hour
Yield: 20 Servings
Ingredients:

- 2 eggs
- 1 teaspoon vanilla extract
- ¼ cup coconut oil, melted
- 1 teaspoon instant coffee
- 6 oz. dark chocolate
- ¼ cup butter
- 2 tablespoons all-purpose flour
- ¼ teaspoon salt
- 2/3 cup white sugar

Directions:

1. Mix the chocolate and butter in a heatproof container and place over a hot water bath. Melt them together until smooth and melted.
2. Mix the eggs and sugar in a container until fluffy and pale. Put in the vanilla and oil and stir lightly. Stir in the coffee.
3. Put in the melted chocolate and stir lightly then fold in the flour and salt.
4. Drop spoonfuls of batter on a baking tray coated with baking paper.
5. Pre-heat the oven and bake at 350F for about ten minutes or until set.
6. *These cookies taste best chilled.*

Nutritional Content of One Serving:
Calories: 124 | Fat: 8.0g | Protein: 1.3g | Carbohydrates: 12.4g

Double Ginger Cookies

Total Time Taken: 1 ¼ hours
Yield: 20 Servings
Ingredients:

- ¼ cup candied ginger, chopped
- ¼ teaspoon salt
- ½ teaspoon baking soda
- ½ teaspoon cinnamon powder
- 1 teaspoon ground ginger
- 1 teaspoon vanilla extract
- 1/3 cup butter, softened
- 2 cups all-purpose flour
- 2 tablespoons golden syrup
- 2/3 cup light brown sugar

Directions:

1. Sift the flour, ginger, cinnamon, salt and baking soda in a container.
2. Mix the butter, sugar, vanilla and syrup in a container until fluffy and pale.
3. Fold in the flour then put in the candied ginger.
4. Drop spoonfuls of batter on a baking sheet coated with baking paper.
5. Pre-heat the oven and bake at 350F for about fifteen minutes or until it rises and looks golden brown.
6. *These cookies taste best chilled.*

Nutritional Content of One Serving:
Calories: 98 | Fat: 3.2g | Protein: 1.4g | Carbohydrates: 16.1g

Dried Cranberry Oatmeal Cookies

Total Time Taken: 1 ¼ hours
Yield: 20 Servings
Ingredients:

- ¼ teaspoon salt
- ½ cup butter, softened, melted
- ½ cup dried cranberries
- ½ cup light brown sugar
- ½ teaspoon cinnamon powder
- ½ teaspoon ground ginger
- 1 cup all-purpose flour
- 1 cup rolled oats
- 1 teaspoon baking soda
- 4 tablespoons golden syrup

Directions:

1. Mix the oats, flour, baking soda, spices, salt and cranberries in a container.
2. Stir in the butter, golden syrup and sugar and mix thoroughly.
3. Make small balls for dough and place the balls on a baking sheet coated with baking paper.
4. Flatten the cookies slightly and preheat your oven and bake at 350F for fifteen minutes or until a golden-brown colour is achieved and fragrant.
5. *These cookies taste best chilled.*

Nutritional Content of One Serving:
Calories: 106 | Fat: 4.9g | Protein: 1.2g | Carbohydrates: 14.5g

Dried Fruit Wholesome Cookies

Total Time Taken: 1 ¼ hours
Yield: 20 Servings
Ingredients:

- ¼ cup applesauce
- ¼ cup coconut oil, melted
- ¼ cup dried apricots, chopped
- ¼ cup dried cranberries
- ¼ cup golden raisins
- ¼ cup rolled oats
- ¼ teaspoon salt

- ½ teaspoon baking soda
- ½ teaspoon cinnamon powder
- 1 ¼ cups whole wheat flour
- 1 egg
- 1 teaspoon vanilla extract

Directions:

1. Mix the coconut oil, applesauce, egg and vanilla and mix thoroughly.
2. Stir in the flour, salt, baking soda and cinnamon then put in the oats and dried fruits.
3. Drop spoonfuls of batter on a baking tray coated with baking paper.
4. Preheat your oven and bake the cookies at 350F for about ten minutes or until a golden-brown colour is achieved and crisp on the edges.
5. *These cookies taste best chilled.*

Nutritional Content of One Serving:

Calories: 68 | Fat: 3.1g | Protein: 1.3g | Carbohydrates: 8.8g

Dried Prune Oatmeal Cookies

Total Time Taken: 1 ¼ hours

Yield: 25 Servings

Ingredients:

- ¼ teaspoon salt
- ½ cup coconut oil, melted
- ½ cup maple syrup
- ½ teaspoon baking soda
- ¾ cup all-purpose flour
- 1 cup dried prunes, chopped
- 1 teaspoon lemon juice
- 1 teaspoon vanilla extract
- 2 cups rolled oats

Directions:

1. Mix the prunes, oats, flour, baking soda and salt in a container.
2. Put in the rest of the ingredients and mix using a spatula.
3. Make small balls of dough and arrange them on a baking sheet coated with baking paper.
4. Preheat your oven and bake the cookies at 350F for about fifteen minutes or until a golden-brown colour is achieved.
5. *These cookies taste best chilled.*

Nutritional Content of One Serving:

Calories: 109 | Fat: 4.9g | Protein: 1.4g | Carbohydrates: 15.9g

Earl Grey Cookies

Total Time Taken: 1 ¼ hours

Yield: 20 Servings

Ingredients:

- ½ cup powdered sugar
- ½ teaspoon salt
- 1 cup butter, softened
- 1 egg
- 1 tablespoon loose Earl grey leaves
- 1 teaspoon baking powder
- 1 teaspoon vanilla extract
- 2 cups all-purpose flour

Directions:

1. Mix the butter and sugar in a container until fluffy and pale.
2. Put in the egg and vanilla and mix thoroughly.
3. Stir in the remaining ingredients and mix using a spatula.
4. Transfer the dough to a floured working surface and roll it into a slim sheet.
5. Cut into small cookies with your cookie cutters and place them on a baking tray coated with baking paper.
6. Pre-heat the oven and bake at 350F for about ten minutes or until a golden-brown colour is achieved on the edges.
7. *These cookies taste best chilled.*

Nutritional Content of One Serving:

Calories: 143 | Fat: 9.6g | Protein: 1.7g | Carbohydrates: 12.7g

Eggless Cookies

Total Time Taken: 1 hour

Yield: 20 Servings

Ingredients:

- ¼ cup whole milk
- ¼ teaspoon salt
- ½ cup butter, melted
- ½ cup dried cranberries
- ½ cup light brown sugar
- ½ teaspoon baking soda
- 1 ½ cups all-purpose flour

Directions:

1. Mix the flour, salt, baking soda and sugar in a container.
2. Stir in the butter and milk and mix using a spatula.
3. Fold in the cranberries then drop spoonfuls of batter on a baking sheet coated with baking paper.
4. Pre-heat the oven and bake at 350F for about fifteen minutes or until a golden-brown colour is achieved on the edges.
5. *These cookies taste best chilled.*

Nutritional Content of One Serving:

Calories: 92 | Fat: 4.8g | Protein: 1.1g | Carbohydrates: 11.1g

Fig and Almond Cookies

Total Time Taken: 1 ¼ hours

Yield: 20 Servings

Ingredients:

- ½ cup butter, softened
- ½ cup ground almonds

- ½ teaspoon baking soda
- ½ teaspoon salt
- 1 ½ cups dried figs, chopped
- 1 ¾ cups all-purpose flour
- 1 cup powdered sugar
- 1 egg
- 1 teaspoon vanilla extract

Directions:

1. Mix the butter, sugar and vanilla in a container until fluffy and pale.
2. Put in the egg and mix thoroughly then fold in the remaining ingredients.
3. Drop spoonfuls of batter on a baking tray coated with baking paper.
4. Pre-heat the oven and bake at 350F for about fifteen minutes or until a golden-brown colour is achieved on the edges and slightly crisp.
5. *These cookies taste best chilled.*

Nutritional Content of One Serving:

Calories: 159 | Fat: 6.3g | Protein: 2.5g | Carbohydrates: 24.4g

Everything-But-The-Kitchen-Sink Cookies

Total Time Taken: 1 ¼ hours

Yield: 20 Servings

Ingredients:

- ¼ cup applesauce
- ¼ cup coconut oil, melted
- ¼ cup dark chocolate chips
- ¼ cup dried apricots, chopped
- ¼ cup dried cranberries
- ¼ cup shredded coconut
- ¼ teaspoon cinnamon powder
- ½ cup walnuts, chopped
- ½ teaspoon ground ginger
- ½ teaspoon salt
- 1 cup rolled oats
- 1 cup whole wheat flour
- 1 egg
- 1 teaspoon vanilla extract
- 2 tablespoons butter, softened

Directions:

1. Mix the coconut oil, butter, vanilla, egg and applesauce in a container.
2. Put in the flour, oats, spices and salt then fold in the walnuts, apricots, cranberries, apricots, chocolate chips and coconut.
3. Drop spoonfuls of batter on baking trays coated with baking paper.
4. Preheat your oven and bake the cookies at 350F for about fifteen minutes or until a golden-brown colour is achieved and crisp on the edges.
5. These cookies taste best chilled.

Nutritional Content of One Serving:

Calories: 109 | Fat: 7.0g | Protein: 2.4g | Carbohydrates: 9.8g

Flourless Peanut Butter Cookies

Total Time Taken: 1 hour

Yield: 30 Servings

Ingredients:

- ½ teaspoon salt
- 1 cup light brown sugar
- 2 cups smooth peanut butter
- 2 eggs

Directions:

1. Combine all the ingredients in a container until the desired smoothness is achieved.
2. Drop spoonfuls of mixture on a baking sheet coated with baking paper.
3. Score the top of each cookie with a fork then preheat your oven and bake the cookies at 350F for about ten minutes.
4. *These cookies taste best chilled.*

Nutritional Content of One Serving:

Calories: 124 | Fat: 9.0g | Protein: 4.7g | Carbohydrates: 8.1g

Four Ingredient Peanut Butter Cookies

Total Time Taken: 1 hour

Yield: 20 Servings

Ingredients:

- 1 cup rolled oats
- 1 cup smooth peanut butter
- 1 egg
- 2/3 cup light brown sugar

Directions:

1. Mix the peanut butter, egg and sugar in a container until creamy then put in the oats.
2. Drop spoonfuls of batter on a baking tray coated with baking paper.
3. Preheat your oven and bake the cookies at 350F for about fifteen minutes or until a golden-brown colour is achieved on the edges.
4. *These cookies taste best chilled.*

Nutritional Content of One Serving:

Calories: 113 | Fat: 7.0g | Protein: 4.1g | Carbohydrates: 10.1g

Fresh Blueberry Cookies

Total Time Taken: 1 ½ hours

Yield: 30 Servings

Ingredients:

- ¼ cup whole milk
- ½ teaspoon baking soda
- ½ teaspoon salt
- 1 cup butter, softened
- 1 cup fresh blueberries
- 1 cup powdered sugar
- 1 egg
- 1 tablespoon lemon zest
- 1 teaspoon vanilla extract
- 2 cups all-purpose flour

Directions:
1. Mix the butter, vanilla and sugar in a container until fluffy and light.
2. Put in the egg, milk and lemon zest and mix thoroughly.
3. Stir in the flour, salt and baking soda and mix using a spatula then fold in the blueberries.
4. Drop spoonfuls of batter on a baking tray covered with parchment paper.
5. Pre-heat the oven and bake at 350F for about thirteen minutes or until a golden-brown colour is achieved on the edges.
6. *These cookies taste best chilled.*

Nutritional Content of One Serving:
Calories: 107 | Fat: 6.5g | Protein: 1.2g | Carbohydrates: 11.2g

Fruity Cookies

Total Time Taken: 1 ½ hours
Yield: 30 Servings
Ingredients:
- 2 tablespoons molasses
- 2 tablespoons golden syrup
- 1 egg
- ¼ cup milk
- 2 cups all-purpose flour
- ¼ teaspoon salt
- 1 teaspoon baking soda
- ½ cup sultanas
- ½ cup dried cranberries
- ½ cup raisins
- ½ cup dried apricots, chopped
- ¼ cup Grand Marnier
- 2/3 cup butter, softened
- 2/3 cup white sugar

Directions:
1. Mix the fruits with Grand Marnier in a container and allow to soak up for about half an hour.
2. Mix the butter, sugar, molasses and golden syrup in a container until pale.
3. Put in the egg and milk and mix thoroughly.
4. Put in the dry ingredients then fold in the fruits.
5. Drop spoonfuls of batter on a baking sheet coated with baking paper and preheat your oven and bake the cookies at 350F for fifteen minutes.
6. Let the cookies cool down before you serve.

Nutritional Content of One Serving:
Calories: 111 | Fat: 4.4g | Protein: 1.3g | Carbohydrates: 15.7g

Fudgy Chocolate Cookies

Total Time Taken: 1 ¼ hours
Yield: 30 Servings
Ingredients:
- ¼ teaspoon salt
- ½ cup butter
- ½ cup light brown sugar
- 1 ½ cups dark chocolate chips
- 1 teaspoon baking powder
- 1 teaspoon vanilla extract
- 2 eggs
- 2 tablespoons white sugar
- 2/3 cup all-purpose flour

Directions:
1. Melt the butter and chocolate in a heatproof container over a hot water bath.
2. Mix the eggs and sugars in a container until fluffy and pale.
3. Stir in the chocolate and mix using a spatula.
4. Fold in the flour, baking powder and salt then drop spoonfuls of batter in a baking sheet coated with baking paper.
5. Preheat your oven and bake the cookies at 350F for about thirteen minutes.
6. *These cookies taste best chilled.*

Nutritional Content of One Serving:
Calories: 82 | Fat: 5.0g | Protein: 1.1g | Carbohydrates: 9.4g

German Chocolate Cookies

Total Time Taken: 1 ¼ hours
Yield: 30 Servings
Ingredients:
- ¼ cup cocoa powder
- ½ cup coconut flakes
- ½ cup dark chocolate chips
- ½ cup white sugar
- ½ teaspoon salt
- 1 cup butter, softened
- 1 cup light brown sugar
- 1 cup pecans, chopped
- 1 teaspoon baking soda
- 2 ¼ cups all-purpose flour
- 2 eggs

Directions:
1. Mix the butter and sugars in a container until pale and creamy.
2. Put in the eggs and mix thoroughly then fold in the flour, cocoa powder, baking soda and salt.
3. Fold in the chocolate chips, coconut flakes and pecans.
4. Drop spoonfuls of batter on baking trays coated with baking paper.
5. Preheat your oven and bake the cookies at 350F for about fifteen minutes or until risen.
6. *These cookies taste best chilled.*

Nutritional Content of One Serving:
Calories: 142 | Fat: 7.9g | Protein: 1.8g | Carbohydrates: 17.2g

Ginger Almond Biscotti

Total Time Taken: 1 ¼ hours
Yield: 20 Servings
Ingredients:

- ¼ teaspoon baking soda
- ½ cup blanched almonds
- ½ cup butter, softened
- ½ teaspoon salt
- ¾ cup white sugar
- 1 teaspoon baking powder
- 1 teaspoon ground ginger
- 1 teaspoon vanilla extract
- 2 cups all-purpose flour
- 2 eggs
- 2 tablespoons dark brown sugar
- 2 tablespoons molasses

Directions:

1. Mix the sugars, molasses, eggs and butter in a container until creamy.
2. Put in the vanilla then fold in the remaining ingredients.
3. Transfer the dough to a baking tray covered with parchment paper and shape it into a log.
4. Preheat your oven and bake the log at 350F for fifteen minutes or until a golden-brown colour is achieved on the edges.
5. When finished, let cool down slightly then cut the log into thin slices and place them back on the baking tray with the cut facing up.
6. Preheat your oven and bake the cookies at 350F for another ten to fifteen minutes.
7. Serve the biscotti chilled.

Nutritional Content of One Serving:
Calories: 145 | Fat: 6.4g | Protein: 2.4g | Carbohydrates: 20.2g

Ginger Butter Cookies

Total Time Taken: 1 ¼ hours
Yield: 20 Servings
Ingredients:

- ¼ teaspoon salt
- ½ cup butter, softened
- ½ teaspoon baking soda
- ½ teaspoon ground cardamom
- ¾ cup light brown sugar
- 1 ½ cups all-purpose flour
- 1 egg
- 1 teaspoon ground ginger
- 1 teaspoon vanilla extract

Directions:

1. Mix the butter and sugar until fluffy and pale. Put in the egg and vanilla and mix thoroughly.
2. Stir in the flour, ginger, cardamom, salt and baking soda.
3. Drop spoonfuls of batter on baking trays coated with baking paper.
4. Preheat your oven and bake the cookies at 350F for about fifteen minutes or until a golden-brown colour is achieved and crisp on the edges.
5. *These cookies taste best chilled.*

Nutritional Content of One Serving:
Calories: 100 | Fat: 4.9g | Protein: 1.3g | Carbohydrates: 12.6g

Ginger Chocolate Oatmeal Cookies

Total Time Taken: 1 ¼ hours
Yield: 30 Servings
Ingredients:

- ¼ teaspoon salt
- ½ teaspoon baking soda
- ½ teaspoon cinnamon powder
- 1 cup all-purpose flour
- 1 cup light brown sugar
- 1 cup rolled oats
- 1 egg
- 1 teaspoon grated ginger
- 2 tablespoons cocoa powder
- 2/3 cup butter, softened

Directions:

1. Mix the butter and sugar until fluffy and creamy. Stir in the egg and mix thoroughly.
2. Put in the rest of the ingredients and mix using a spatula.
3. Drop spoonfuls of batter on a baking sheet coated with baking paper.
4. Pre-heat the oven and bake at 350F for fifteen minutes.
5. *These cookies taste best chilled.*

Nutritional Content of One Serving:
Calories: 83 | Fat: 4.5g | Protein: 1.1g | Carbohydrates: 10.0g

Ginger Quinoa Cookies

Total Time Taken: 1 ¼ hours
Yield: 30 Servings
Ingredients:

- ¼ cup quinoa flakes
- ¼ cup quinoa flour
- ¼ teaspoon salt
- ½ cup almond flour
- ½ cup coconut oil, melted
- ½ cup light brown sugar
- ½ teaspoon baking soda
- ½ teaspoon cinnamon powder
- ½ teaspoon ground ginger
- 1 cup all-purpose flour
- 1 egg
- 2 tablespoons butter, softened
- 2 tablespoons molasses

Directions:

1. Mix the coconut oil and butter, molasses and sugar in a container until creamy and fluffy.

2. Put in the egg and mix thoroughly.
3. Stir in the remaining ingredients then drop spoonfuls of batter on a baking sheet coated with baking paper.
4. Preheat your oven and bake the cookies at 350F for about fifteen minutes or until a golden-brown colour is achieved on the edges.
5. These cookies taste best chilled.

Nutritional Content of One Serving:
Calories: 79 | Fat: 5.0g | Protein: 1.2g | Carbohydrates: 7.6g

Gingerbread Cookies

Total Time Taken: 1 ¼ hours
Yield: 30 Servings
Ingredients:

- ¼ teaspoon salt
- ½ cup golden syrup
- ½ cup white sugar
- ½ teaspoon ground cardamom
- 1 cup butter, softened
- 1 egg
- 1 teaspoon baking soda
- 1 teaspoon cinnamon powder
- 1 teaspoon ground ginger
- 2 cups all-purpose flour
- 2 tablespoons dark molasses

Directions:
1. Mix the butter, golden syrup, sugar and molasses in a container until fluffy and pale.
2. Put in the egg and mix thoroughly then fold in the flour, spices, baking soda and salt.
3. Make small balls of dough and arrange them on a baking sheet coated with baking paper.
4. Pre-heat the oven and bake at 350F for fifteen minutes or until it is aromatic and appears golden.
5. *These cookies taste best chilled.*

Nutritional Content of One Serving:
Calories: 119 | Fat: 6.4g | Protein: 1.1g | Carbohydrates: 15.0g

Gingerbread Cookies

Total Time Taken: 1 ¼ hours
Yield: 20 Servings
Ingredients:

- ¼ cup molasses
- ¼ teaspoon salt
- ½ cup butter, softened
- ½ cup ground almonds
- ½ cup light brown sugar
- ½ teaspoon baking soda
- ½ teaspoon cinnamon powder
- ½ teaspoon ground cloves
- ½ teaspoon ground ginger
- 1 egg
- 2 cups all-purpose flour

Directions:
1. Mix the butter, molasses and sugar in a container until pale and creamy.
2. Put in the egg and mix thoroughly then mix in the rest of the ingredients.
3. Make small balls of dough and place them on a baking tray coated with baking paper.
4. Preheat your oven and bake the cookies at 350F for about thirteen minutes or until aromatic, risen and golden.
5. *These cookies taste best chilled.*

Nutritional Content of One Serving:
Calories: 129 | Fat: 6.2g | Protein: 2.1g | Carbohydrates: 16.8g

Gingersnap Cookies

Total Time Taken: 1 hour
Yield: 20 Servings
Ingredients:

- ¼ cup molasses
- ¼ teaspoon salt
- ½ teaspoon baking powder
- ½ teaspoon cinnamon powder
- ¾ cup canola oil
- ¾ cup light brown sugar
- 1 egg
- 1 teaspoon baking soda
- 1 teaspoon ground ginger
- 2 cups all-purpose flour

Directions:
1. Mix the oil, molasses and sugar in a container.
2. Put in the egg and stir until creamy and pale.
3. Fold in the remaining ingredients then form small balls and place them on baking trays coated with baking paper.
4. Preheat your oven and bake the cookies at 350F for about fifteen minutes or until crisp and fragrant.
5. *These cookies taste best chilled.*

Nutritional Content of One Serving:
Calories: 154 | Fat: 8.5g | Protein: 1.6g | Carbohydrates: 18.1g

Gooey Chocolate Cherry Cookies

Total Time Taken: 1 hour
Yield: 20 Servings
Ingredients:

- ¼ cup white sugar
- ½ cup butter, melted
- ½ cup dark chocolate chips
- ½ cup glace cherries, halved
- ½ cup muscovado sugar
- 1 ½ cups all-purpose flour
- 1 egg

- 2 tablespoons cocoa powder

Directions:

1. Combine all the ingredients in a container using a spatula.
2. Drop spoonfuls of batter on a baking tray coated with baking paper.
3. Pre-heat the oven and bake at 350F for about ten minutes.
4. *These cookies taste best chilled.*

Nutritional Content of One Serving:

Calories: 128 | Fat: 5.8g | Protein: 1.7g | Carbohydrates: 18.2g

Hazelnut Chocolate Chip Cookies

Total Time Taken: 1 ¼ hours

Yield: 30 Servings

Ingredients:

- ¼ cup sour cream
- ½ cup mini chocolate chip cookies
- ½ cup rolled oats, ground
- ½ teaspoon salt
- 1 cup butter, softened
- 1 cup ground hazelnuts
- 1 cup light brown sugar
- 1 egg
- 1 teaspoon baking powder
- 1 teaspoon vanilla extract
- 2 cups all-purpose flour

Directions:

1. Mix the butter and sugar in a container until creamy and fluffy.
2. Put in the egg and vanilla and sour cream and mix thoroughly the mix in the dry ingredients and chocolate chips.
3. Transfer the dough to a floured working surface and roll it into a slim sheet.
4. Cut into small cookies with your cookie cutters and place the cookies on baking trays coated with baking paper.
5. Preheat your oven and bake the cookies at 350F for about fifteen minutes or until a golden-brown colour is achieved on the edges.
6. *These cookies taste best chilled.*

Nutritional Content of One Serving:

Calories: 135 | Fat: 8.6g | Protein: 1.8g | Carbohydrates: 13.1g

Healthy Banana Cookies

Total Time Taken: 1 hour

Yield: 25 Servings

Ingredients:

- ¼ cup coconut flakes
- ¼ cup coconut oil, melted
- ¼ cup dried cranberries
- ¼ cup dried mango, chopped
- 1 cup dates, pitted and chopped
- 2 cups rolled oats
- 4 ripe bananas, mashed

Directions:

1. Mix the bananas and oil then mix in the rest of the ingredients.
2. Drop spoonfuls of batter on baking trays coated with baking paper.
3. Pre-heat the oven and bake at 350F for about fifteen minutes or until a golden-brown colour is achieved.
4. *These cookies taste best chilled.*

Nutritional Content of One Serving:

Calories: 114 | Fat: 3.0g | Protein: 1.3g | Carbohydrates: 21.8g

Honey Cornflake Cookies

Total Time Taken: 1 ¼ hours

Yield: 20 Servings

Ingredients:

- ¼ teaspoon salt
- ½ cup honey
- ½ cup light brown sugar
- 1 ¾ cups all-purpose flour
- 1 cup cornflakes
- 1 egg
- 1 teaspoon baking powder
- 1 teaspoon vanilla extract
- 2 tablespoons pine nuts
- 2/3 cup butter, softened

Directions:

1. Mix the butter, honey and sugar in a container.
2. Stir in the egg and vanilla and mix thoroughly then fold in the remaining ingredients.
3. Drop spoonfuls of batter on a baking sheet coated with baking paper.
4. Pre-heat the oven and bake at 350F for about fifteen minutes or until a golden-brown colour is achieved on the edges.
5. *These cookies taste best chilled.*

Nutritional Content of One Serving:

Calories: 148 | Fat: 7.1g | Protein: 1.7g | Carbohydrates: 20.4g

Honey Lemon Cookies

Total Time Taken: 1 ¼ hours

Yield: 40 Servings

Ingredients:

- ¼ cup honey
- ½ teaspoon salt
- ¾ cup white sugar
- 1 cup butter, softened
- 1 egg
- 1 lemon, zested and juiced
- 1 teaspoon baking soda
- 3 cups all-purpose flour

Directions:

1. Sift the flour, baking soda and salt in a container.
2. In a separate container, combine the butter, sugar and honey and mix thoroughly.
3. Stir in the lemon zest and juice, as well as the egg.
4. Fold in the flour mixture then roll the dough into a slim sheet over a floured working surface.
5. Cut the cookies using a cookie cutter of your choices.
6. Put the cookies in the preheated oven at 350F for about fifteen minutes or until a golden-brown colour is achieved on the edges.
7. *These cookies taste best chilled.*

Nutritional Content of One Serving:

Calories: 97 | Fat: 4.8g | Protein: 1.2g | Carbohydrates: 12.8g

Icing Decorated Cookies

Total Time Taken: 1 ¼ hours
Yield: 20 Servings
Ingredients:
Cookies:

- ¼ teaspoon salt
- ½ cup butter, softened
- ½ cup powdered sugar
- ½ teaspoon baking powder
- 1 ½ cups all-purpose flour
- 1 egg yolk

Icing:

- ¼ teaspoon vanilla extract
- 1 cup powdered sugar
- 1 egg white

Directions:

1. For the cookies, combine the butter and sugar in a container until fluffy and pale.
2. Put in the egg yolk and mix thoroughly then fold in the flour, salt and baking powder.
3. Transfer the dough to a floured working surface and roll the dough into slim sheet.
4. Cut into small cookies with a cookie cutter and arrange the cookies on a baking tray coated with baking paper.
5. Preheat your oven and bake the cookies at 350F for about ten minutes or until a golden-brown colour is achieved on the edges.
6. For the icing, combine the sugar, egg white and vanilla in a container.
7. Spoon the icing in a small piping bag and garnish the chilled cookies with it.

Nutritional Content of One Serving:

Calories: 114 | Fat: 4.9g | Protein: 1.3g | Carbohydrates: 16.2g

Layered Chocolate Chip Cookies

Total Time Taken: 1 ¼ hours
Yield: 30 Servings
Ingredients:

- ¼ cup dark brown sugar
- ½ teaspoon salt
- ¾ cup light brown sugar
- 1 cup butter, softened
- 1 cup dark chocolate chips
- 1 teaspoon baking soda
- 1 teaspoon vanilla extract
- 2 ¼ cups all-purpose flour
- 2 eggs

Directions:

1. Mix the butter and sugars in a container until fluffy and pale.
2. Put in the eggs and mix thoroughly then fold in the remaining ingredients.
3. Drop spoonfuls of batter on baking trays covered with parchment paper.
4. Preheat your oven and bake the cookies at 350F for about thirteen minutes or until a golden-brown colour is achieved.
5. *These cookies taste best chilled.*

Nutritional Content of One Serving:

Calories: 130 | Fat: 7.6g | Protein: 1.7g | Carbohydrates: 14.6g

Lemon Poppy Seed Cookies

Total Time Taken: 1 hour
Yield: 20 Servings
Ingredients:

- ¼ cup butter, softened
- ¼ cup coconut oil
- ¼ cup cornstarch
- ¼ teaspoon salt
- ½ teaspoon baking soda
- 1 cup all-purpose flour
- 1 egg
- 1 tablespoon lemon zest
- 2 tablespoons lemon juice
- 2 tablespoons poppy seeds
- 2/3 cup white sugar

Directions:

1. Mix the butter, coconut oil and sugar in a container until fluffy and pale.
2. Put in the egg, lemon zest and lemon juice and mix thoroughly.
3. Fold in the remaining ingredients and mix using a spatula.
4. Drop spoonfuls of batter on baking trays coated with baking paper.
5. Preheat your oven and bake the cookies at 350F for about fifteen minutes or until a golden-brown colour is achieved or until a golden-brown colour is achieved on the edges.
6. *These cookies taste best chilled.*

Nutritional Content of One Serving:
Calories: 106 | Fat: 5.7g | Protein: 1.1g | Carbohydrates: 13.2g

Lemon Ricotta Cookies

Total Time Taken: 2 hours
Yield: 40 Servings
Ingredients:

- ¼ cup butter, softened
- ½ teaspoon salt
- 1 cup ricotta cheese
- 1 cup white sugar
- 1 tablespoon lemon zest
- 1 teaspoon baking powder
- 2 eggs
- 2 tablespoons lemon juice 2 ½ cups all-purpose flour

Directions:

1. Mix the cheese, sugar, eggs and butter in a container until creamy.
2. Put in the lemon zest and lemon juice then fold in the flour, salt and baking powder.
3. Drop spoonfuls of baking batter on a baking tray covered with parchment paper.
4. Preheat your oven and bake the cookies at 350F for about fifteen minutes or until a golden-brown colour is achieved on the edges.
5. *These cookies taste best chilled.*

Nutritional Content of One Serving:
Calories: 69 | Fat: 1.9g | Protein: 1.8g | Carbohydrates: 11.4g

Lemony Lavender Cookies

Total Time Taken: 1 ¼ hours
Yield: 25 Servings
Ingredients:

- ½ cup butter, softened
- ½ cup white sugar
- ½ teaspoon baking soda
- ½ teaspoon salt
- 1 cup all-purpose flour
- 1 cup almond flour
- 1 egg
- 1 tablespoon lemon zest
- 1 teaspoon lavender buds
- 2 tablespoons honey

Directions:

1. Mix the butter, honey, egg, lemon zest, sugar and lavender in a container until pale and light.
2. Put in the rest of the ingredients and mix using a spatula.
3. Drop spoonfuls of batter on a baking tray coated with baking paper.
4. Preheat your oven and bake the cookies at 350F for about fifteen minutes or until a golden-brown colour is achieved on the edges.
5. *These cookies taste best chilled.*

Nutritional Content of One Serving:
Calories: 82 | Fat: 4.5g | Protein: 1.1g | Carbohydrates: 9.9g

Lentil Cookies

Total Time Taken: 1 ¼ hours
Yield: 30 Servings
Ingredients:

- ¼ teaspoon salt
- ½ cup butter, melted
- ½ cup walnuts, chopped
- ½ teaspoon baking powder
- ½ teaspoon cinnamon powder
- ½ teaspoon ground ginger
- ¾ cup light brown sugar
- 1 ½ cups all-purpose flour
- 1 egg
- 1 teaspoon vanilla extract
- 4 oz. lentil, cooked and pureed

Directions:

1. Mix the lentil puree, butter, egg, vanilla and sugar in a container until creamy and light.
2. Put in the rest of the ingredients and mix thoroughly.
3. Make small balls of mixture and place them on a baking tray coated with baking paper.
4. Preheat your oven and bake the cookies at 350F for about fifteen minutes or until a golden-brown colour is achieved and fragrant.
5. *These cookies taste best chilled.*

Nutritional Content of One Serving:
Calories: 93 | Fat: 4.5g | Protein: 2.3g | Carbohydrates: 10.9g

M&M Cookies

Total Time Taken: 1 ¼ hours
Yield: 30 Servings
Ingredients:

- 1 cup butter, softened
- 2/3 cup light brown sugar
- 2 eggs
- 2 cups all-purpose flour
- 1 teaspoon baking powder
- ¼ teaspoon salt
- 1 cup M&M candies

Directions:

1. Mix the butter and sugar in a container until creamy and fluffy.
2. Stir in the eggs, one at a time, then put in the flour, baking powder and salt.
3. Fold in the candies then drop spoonfuls of batter on a baking tray coated with baking paper.
4. Preheat your oven and bake the cookies at 350F for fifteen minutes or until a golden-brown colour is achieved on the edges.

5. *These cookies taste best chilled.*

Nutritional Content of One Serving:

Calories: 102 | Fat: 6.5g | Protein: 1.3g | Carbohydrates: 9.8g

Macadamia Cookies

Total Time Taken: 1 ¼ hours

Yield: 20 Servings

Ingredients:

- ¼ cup golden syrup
- ¼ cup light brown sugar
- ½ cup butter, softened
- ½ cup shredded coconut
- ½ teaspoon salt
- 1 cup all-purpose flour
- 1 cup rolled oats
- 1 teaspoon baking powder
- 2/3 cup macadamia nuts, chopped

Directions:

1. Mix the oats, flour, baking powder, salt, coconut and macadamia nuts in a container.
2. Mix the butter and syrup and sugar in a container until creamy and pale.
3. Fold in the remaining ingredients then drop spoonfuls of batter on a baking sheet coated with baking paper.
4. Pre-heat the oven and bake at 350F for about fifteen minutes or until a golden-brown colour is achieved on the edges.
5. *These cookies taste best chilled.*

Nutritional Content of One Serving:

Calories: 137 | Fat: 9.0g | Protein: 1.7g | Carbohydrates: 13.5g

Mango Crunch Cookies

Total Time Taken: 1 ¼ hours

Yield: 20 Servings

Ingredients:

- ¼ cup white sugar
- ¼ teaspoon salt
- ½ cup butter, softened
- ½ teaspoon baking soda
- 1 ½ cups all-purpose flour
- 1 cup dried mango, chopped
- 1 egg
- 1 teaspoon vanilla extract

Directions:

1. Mix the butter, sugar and egg in a container until creamy. Put in the vanilla and mix thoroughly then fold in the flour, salt and baking soda.
2. Put in the mango and mix using a spatula.
3. Drop spoonfuls of batter on a baking tray coated with baking paper.
4. Pre-heat the oven and bake at 350F for about fifteen minutes or until a golden-brown colour is achieved on the edges.

5. *These cookies taste best chilled.*

Nutritional Content of One Serving:

Calories: 95 | Fat: 5.0g | Protein: 1.4g | Carbohydrates: 11.5g

Maple Flavored Cookies

Total Time Taken: 1 ¼ hours

Yield: 30 Servings

Ingredients:

- ½ cup butter, softened
- 1 teaspoon vanilla extract
- 1 egg
- ½ cup maple syrup
- 2 cups all-purpose flour
- ¼ teaspoon salt
- 1 teaspoon baking powder
- 1 cup walnuts, chopped
- 1/2 cup light brown sugar

Directions:

1. Mix the butter, sugar and maple syrup in a container until fluffy and creamy.
2. Put in the vanilla and eggs and mix thoroughly then mix in the rest of the ingredients.
3. Drop spoonfuls of batter on baking trays coated with baking paper.
4. Preheat your oven and bake the cookies at 350F for about fifteen minutes or until a golden-brown colour is achieved on the edges.
5. *These cookies taste best chilled.*

Nutritional Content of One Serving:

Calories: 109 | Fat: 5.8g | Protein: 2.1g | Carbohydrates: 12.8g

Maple Sesame Cookies

Total Time Taken: 1 ½ hours

Yield: 25 Servings

Ingredients:

- ¼ cup sesame seeds
- ¼ teaspoon salt
- ½ cup butter, softened
- ½ cup maple syrup
- 1 ½ cups all-purpose flour
- 1 egg
- 1 teaspoon baking powder
- 2 tablespoons dark brown sugar

Directions:

1. Mix the butter, maple syrup and egg in a container until creamy and pale.
2. Stir in the sugar and mix thoroughly then put in the flour, salt, baking powder and sesame seeds.
3. Spoon the batter in a plastic wrap and shape it into a log. Put it in your freezer for about half an hour.

4. Take out of the freezer and cut into thin slices. Position the slices on a baking sheet coated with baking paper with the cut facing up.
5. Pre-heat the oven and bake at 350F for about ten minutes or until mildly golden-brown on the edges.
6. *These cookies taste best chilled.*

Nutritional Content of One Serving:

Calories: 90 | Fat: 4.6g | Protein: 1.3g | Carbohydrates: 11.1g

Marshmallow Chocolate Chip Cookies

Total Time Taken: 1 ¼ hours

Yield: 20 Servings

Ingredients:

- ¼ teaspoon salt
- ½ cup butter, softened
- ½ cup cornflakes
- ½ cup dark chocolate chips
- ½ teaspoon baking soda
- ¾ cup light brown sugar
- 1 ½ cups all-purpose flour
- 1 cup mini marshmallows
- 1 teaspoon vanilla extract
- 2 tablespoons coconut oil
- 2 tablespoons whole milk

Directions:

1. Mix the butter, coconut oil, sugar and vanilla in a container until pale and fluffy.
2. Stir in the milk then put in the flour, baking soda and salt then fold in the cornflakes, chocolate chips and marshmallows.
3. Drop spoonfuls of batter on a baking sheet coated with baking paper.
4. Preheat your oven and bake the cookies at 350F for about fifteen minutes or until a golden-brown colour is achieved on the edges.
5. *These cookies taste best chilled.*

Nutritional Content of One Serving:

Calories: 130 | Fat: 6.9g | Protein: 1.3g | Carbohydrates: 16.3g

Milky Cookies

Total Time Taken: 1 ¼ hours

Yield: 30 Servings

Ingredients:

- ¼ cup milk powder
- ¼ cup whole milk
- ¼ teaspoon salt
- 1 cup butter, softened
- 1 cup white sugar
- 1 teaspoon baking powder
- 1 teaspoon lemon zest
- 1 teaspoon vanilla extract
- 2 cups all-purpose flour
- 2 egg yolks

Directions:

1. Mix the butter, sugar, vanilla and lemon zest in a container until fluffy and pale.
2. Put in the egg yolks and milk and mix thoroughly then mix in the flour, milk powder, baking powder and salt.
3. Drop spoonfuls of batter on a baking tray coated with baking paper.
4. Pre-heat the oven and bake at 350F for about fifteen minutes or until a golden-brown colour is achieved on the edges.
5. Let the cookies cool before you serve.

Nutritional Content of One Serving:

Calories: 119 | Fat: 6.6g | Protein: 1.6g | Carbohydrates: 13.8g

Minty Chocolate Cookies

Total Time Taken: 1 ¼ hours

Yield: 20 Servings

Ingredients:

- ¼ cup cocoa powder
- ¼ teaspoon salt
- ½ cup butter, softened
- ½ cup white sugar
- 1 ¼ cups all-purpose flour
- 1 egg
- 1 teaspoon baking powder
- 1 teaspoon peppermint extract
- 1 teaspoon vanilla extract
- 2 tablespoons honey

Directions:

1. Mix the butter, sugar, honey, peppermint and vanilla in a container until fluffy and pale.
2. Put in the egg and mix thoroughly then fold in the remaining ingredients.
3. Drop spoonfuls of batter on a baking sheet coated with baking paper.
4. Preheat your oven and bake the cookies at 350F for about fifteen minutes or until it rises completely and is aromatic.
5. *These cookies taste best chilled.*

Nutritional Content of One Serving:

Calories: 101 | Fat: 5.0g | Protein: 1.4g | Carbohydrates: 13.5g

Minty Chocolate Cookies

Total Time Taken: 1 ¼ hours

Yield: 20 Servings

Ingredients:

- ¼ cup cocoa powder
- ¼ teaspoon salt
- ½ cup dark chocolate chips
- ¾ cup butter, softened
- 1 1/4 cups all-purpose flour
- 1 cup light brown sugar
- 1 egg

- 1 teaspoon baking powder
- 1 teaspoon peppermint extract
- 1 teaspoon vanilla extract
- 2 tablespoons milk

Directions:

1. Mix the butter, sugar and vanilla in a container until creamy and pale.
2. Put in the milk, peppermint extract and egg and mix thoroughly then fold in the remaining ingredients.
3. Drop spoonfuls of batter on baking trays coated with baking paper.
4. Preheat your oven and bake the cookies at 350F for about thirteen minutes or until aromatic.
5. *These cookies taste best chilled.*

Nutritional Content of One Serving:

Calories: 139 | Fat: 8.2g | Protein: 1.6g | Carbohydrates: 15.9g

Molasses Cookies

Total Time Taken: 1 ½ hours

Yield: 20 Servings

Ingredients:

- ¼ teaspoon salt
- ½ cup butter, softened
- ½ cup light brown sugar
- 1 ½ cups all-purpose flour
- 1 egg
- 1 teaspoon baking powder
- 1 teaspoon vanilla extract
- 4 tablespoons dark molasses

Directions:

1. Mix the butter, molasses and sugar in a container until creamy and fluffy.
2. Put in the egg and vanilla and mix thoroughly.
3. Fold in the remaining ingredients then drop spoonfuls of batter on a baking tray coated with baking paper.
4. Preheat your oven and bake the cookies at 350F for about fifteen minutes or until aromatic and crunchy.
5. *These cookies taste best chilled.*

Nutritional Content of One Serving:

Calories: 104 | Fat: 4.9g | Protein: 1.3g | Carbohydrates: 13.9g

Molten Chocolate Cookies

Total Time Taken: 1 hour

Yield: 20 Servings

Ingredients:

- ¼ cup cocoa powder
- ¼ cup white sugar
- ¼ teaspoon salt
- ½ teaspoon baking soda
- 1 ¾ cups all-purpose flour
- 1 cup light brown sugar
- 1 egg
- 1 egg yolk
- 2/3 cup butter, melted

Directions:

1. Mix the butter, sugars, egg and egg yolk in container until creamy and fluffy.
2. Put in the rest of the ingredients then drop large spoonfuls of batter on a baking sheet coated with baking paper.
3. Pre-heat the oven and bake at 350F for about twelve minutes.
4. **These cookies taste best chilled.**

Nutritional Content of One Serving:

Calories: 139 | Fat: 6.8g | Protein: 1.8g | Carbohydrates: 18.6g

Monster Cookie Recipes

Total Time Taken: 1 ¼ hours

Yield: 30 Servings

Ingredients:

- ¼ cup white sugar
- ½ cup butter, softened
- ½ cup M&M candies
- ½ cup mini marshmallows
- ½ cup pecans, chopped
- ½ cup smooth peanut butter
- ½ cup walnuts, chopped
- ½ teaspoon salt
- ¾ cup light brown sugar
- 1 teaspoon baking soda
- 1 teaspoon vanilla extract
- 2 ¼ cups all-purpose flour
- 2 eggs

Directions:

1. Mix the butter, peanut butter and sugars in a container. Put in the vanilla and eggs and mix thoroughly.
2. Fold in the flour, salt and baking soda then put in the remaining ingredients.
3. Drop spoonfuls of batter on a baking tray covered with parchment paper.
4. Preheat your oven and bake the cookies at 350F for about fifteen minutes or until a golden-brown colour is achieved on the edges.
5. *These cookies taste best chilled.*

Nutritional Content of One Serving:

Calories: 149 | Fat: 7.2g | Protein: 3.2g | Carbohydrates: 18.9g

Muesli Cookies

Total Time Taken: 1 ¼ hours

Yield: 20 Servings

Ingredients:

- ¼ teaspoon salt
- ½ cup butter, softened

- ½ cup white chocolate chips
- ½ cup white sugar
- 1 cup all-purpose flour
- 1 cup muesli
- 1 egg
- 1 teaspoon baking powder

Directions:

1. Mix the butter and sugar until fluffy and creamy. Put in the egg and mix thoroughly.
2. Stir in the flour, baking powder and salt then put in the muesli and chocolate chips.
3. Drop spoonfuls of batter on a baking sheet coated with baking paper.
4. Preheat your oven and bake the cookies at 350F for fifteen minutes or until a golden-brown colour is achieved on the edges.
5. *These cookies taste best chilled.*

Nutritional Content of One Serving:

Calories: 124 | Fat: 6.5g | Protein: 1.6g | Carbohydrates: 15.6g

Nutty Cookies

Total Time Taken: 1 hour

Yield: 20 Servings

Ingredients:

- ¼ cup white sugar
- ¼ teaspoon salt
- ½ cup almond butter
- ½ cup ground cashew nuts
- ½ cup ground walnuts
- ½ cup light brown sugar
- ½ teaspoon baking soda
- 1 ¼ cups all-purpose flour
- 1 egg
- 1 teaspoon vanilla extract

Directions:

1. Mix the almond butter and sugars in a container until pale and light. Put in the egg and vanilla and mix thoroughly.
2. Stir in the remaining ingredients then drop spoonfuls of batter on a baking tray coated with baking paper.
3. Preheat your oven and bake the cookies at 350F for about fifteen minutes or until crisp and golden brown.
4. Serve Chilled or store them in an airtight container.

Nutritional Content of One Serving:

Calories: 138 | Fat: 7.6g | Protein: 3.9g | Carbohydrates: 14.6g

Oatmeal Cookies

Total Time Taken: 1 hour

Yield: 30 Servings

Ingredients:

- ½ cup dried cranberries
- ½ cup light brown sugar
- ½ teaspoon baking soda
- ½ teaspoon salt
- ¾ cup butter, softened
- 1 ½ cups all-purpose flour
- 1 cup pecans, chopped
- 1 cup rolled oats
- 1 egg
- 1 teaspoon vanilla extract
- 2 tablespoons dark brown sugar

Directions:

1. Mix the butter and sugars in a container until fluffy and creamy.
2. Stir in the egg and vanilla and mix thoroughly.
3. Fold in the remaining ingredients.
4. Drop spoonfuls of batter on a baking sheet coated with baking paper.
5. Preheat your oven and bake the cookies at 350F for fifteen minutes or until it rises significantly and seems golden.
6. Let the cookies cool in the pan before you serve.

Nutritional Content of One Serving:

Calories: 92 | Fat: 5.3g | Protein: 1.3g | Carbohydrates: 9.8g

Oatmeal Raisins Cookies

Total Time Taken: 2 hours

Yield: 20 Servings

Ingredients:

- ¼ cup brandy
- ¼ teaspoon salt
- ½ cup golden raisins
- ½ cup light brown sugar
- 1 cup rolled oats
- 1 cup whole wheat flour
- 1 egg
- 1 teaspoon baking powder
- 1 teaspoon vanilla extract
- 2/3 cup butter, softened

Directions:

1. Mix the raisins and brandy in a container and let them soak up for an hour.
2. Mix the butter and sugar in a container until fluffy and pale.
3. Put in the egg and vanilla and mix thoroughly.
4. Put in the flour, salt, baking powder and oats then fold in the raisins.
5. Drop spoonfuls of batter on a baking sheet coated with baking paper.
6. Pre-heat the oven and bake at 350F for fifteen minutes or until the edges turn golden brown.
7. *These cookies taste best chilled.*

Nutritional Content of One Serving:

Calories: 124 | Fat: 6.7g | Protein: 1.6g | Carbohydrates: 14.1g

Olive Oil Chocolate Chip Cookies

Total Time Taken: 1 ¼ hours
Yield: 30 Servings
Ingredients:

- ¼ cup butter, softened
- ¼ cup white sugar
- ¼ teaspoon salt
- ½ cup dark chocolate chips
- ½ cup light brown sugar
- ½ cup olive oil
- ½ cup white chocolate chips
- 1 egg
- 1 teaspoon baking powder
- 1 teaspoon vanilla extract
- 2 cups all-purpose flour

Directions:

1. Mix the oil, butter and sugars in a container until creamy and fluffy.
2. Put in the vanilla and egg and mix thoroughly.
3. Fold in the flour, salt and baking powder, then put in the chocolate chips.
4. Drop spoonfuls of batter on a baking sheet coated with baking paper.
5. Pre-heat the oven and bake at 350F for about fifteen minutes or until a golden-brown colour is achieved on the edges.
6. *These cookies taste best chilled.*

Nutritional Content of One Serving:
Calories: 115 | Fat: 6.6g | Protein: 1.4g | Carbohydrates: 13.5g

Orange Passionfruit Cookies

Total Time Taken: 1 ¼ hours
Yield: 20 Servings
Ingredients:

- 1 teaspoon vanilla extract
- 1 egg
- 1 teaspoon orange zest
- Juice from 2 passionfruits
- 2 cups all-purpose flour
- ¼ teaspoon salt
- 1 teaspoon baking powder
- 2/3 cup butter, softened
- 2/3 cup white sugar

Directions:

1. Mix the butter, sugar and vanilla until creamy and fluffy.
2. Put in the egg, orange zest and passionfruit juice then mix in the dry ingredients.
3. Drop spoonfuls of batter on a baking tray coated with baking paper.
4. Preheat your oven and bake the cookies at 350F for about fifteen minutes or until the edges turn golden brown.
5. *These cookies taste best chilled.*

Nutritional Content of One Serving:
Calories: 129 | Fat: 6.5g | Protein: 1.6g | Carbohydrates: 16.4g

Orange Pistachio Cookies

Total Time Taken: 1 ¼ hours
Yield: 20 Servings
Ingredients:

- ¼ cup powdered sugar
- ¼ teaspoon salt
- ½ cup almond flour
- ½ cup butter, softened
- ½ cup ground pistachio
- ½ teaspoon baking soda
- 1 cup all-purpose flour
- 1 egg
- 1 teaspoon orange zest
- 2 tablespoons fresh orange juice

Directions:

1. Mix the almonds and pistachio in a container.
2. Mix the butter with sugar until fluffy and pale.
3. Stir in the egg, orange juice and orange zest.
4. Stir in the flour, salt, baking soda and pistachio mixture.
5. Drop spoonfuls of batter on a baking sheet coated with baking paper.
6. Preheat your oven and bake the cookies at 350F for about fifteen minutes or until a golden-brown colour is achieved on the edges.
7. *These cookies taste best chilled.*

Nutritional Content of One Serving:
Calories: 88 | Fat: 5.7g | Protein: 1.4g | Carbohydrates: 8.0g

Orange Poppy Seed Cookies

Total Time Taken: 1 ¼ hours
Yield: 20 Servings
Ingredients:

- ¼ teaspoon salt
- ½ cup butter, softened
- ½ cup white sugar
- ½ teaspoon baking powder
- 1 ½ cups all-purpose flour
- 1 egg
- 1 tablespoon orange zest
- 1 tablespoon poppy seeds

Directions:

1. Mix the butter and sugar in a container until fluffy and creamy.

2. Put in the egg and orange zest and mix thoroughly then fold in the flour, salt, baking powder and poppy seeds.
3. Drop spoonfuls of batter on a baking tray coated with baking paper.
4. Preheat your oven and bake the cookies at 350F for about fifteen minutes or until a golden-brown colour is achieved on the edges.
5. *These cookies taste best chilled.*

Nutritional Content of One Serving:
Calories: 100 | Fat: 5.1g | Protein: 1.4g | Carbohydrates: 12.4g

Orange Pumpkin Cookies

Total Time Taken: 1 hour
Yield: 20 Servings
Ingredients:

- ¼ teaspoon salt
- ½ cup almond flour
- ½ cup butter, softened
- ½ cup powdered sugar
- ½ cup pumpkin puree
- 1 ½ cups all-purpose flour
- 1 orange, zested and juiced
- 1 teaspoon baking powder

Directions:

1. Mix the butter and sugar in a container until pale and creamy.
2. Put in the orange zest and juice, as well as the pumpkin puree and mix thoroughly.
3. Fold in the flour, almond flour, salt and baking powder then drop spoonfuls of batter on a baking tray coated with baking paper.
4. Preheat your oven and bake the cookies at 350F for about fifteen minutes or until a golden-brown colour is achieved or until a golden-brown colour is achieved and fragrant.
5. *These cookies taste best chilled.*

Nutritional Content of One Serving:
Calories: 97 | Fat: 5.1g | Protein: 1.3g | Carbohydrates: 12.0g

Outrageous Chocolate Cookies

Total Time Taken: 1 ¼ hours
Yield: 20 Servings
Ingredients:

- ¼ cup butter, softened
- ¼ cup coconut oil
- ½ cup dark chocolate chips
- ½ teaspoon salt
- ¾ cup light brown sugar
- 1 cup all-purpose flour
- 1 teaspoon baking powder
- 1 teaspoon vanilla extract
- 2 eggs
- 4 oz. dark chocolate, melted

Directions:

1. Mix the butter, coconut oil and sugar in a container until pale and creamy.
2. Mix the eggs, one at a time, then mix in the chocolate and vanilla.
3. Fold in the flour, salt and baking powder, as well as the chocolate chips.
4. Drop spoonfuls of batter on a baking tray coated with baking paper.
5. Pre-heat the oven and bake at 350F for about fifteen minutes or until a golden-brown colour is achieved and it rises significantly.
6. *These cookies taste best chilled.*

Nutritional Content of One Serving:
Calories: 139 | Fat: 8.0g | Protein: 1.9g | Carbohydrates: 15.7g

Peanut Butter Chocolate Cookies

Total Time Taken: 1 hour
Yield: 20 Servings
Ingredients:

- ¼ cup butter, softened
- ¼ cup smooth peanut butter
- ¼ teaspoon salt
- ½ cup chocolate chips
- ½ cup light brown sugar
- ½ teaspoon baking powder
- ½ teaspoon baking soda
- 1 cup all-purpose flour
- 1 egg

Directions:

1. Mix the butters and sugar in a container until creamy and fluffy.
2. Stir in the egg and mix thoroughly.
3. Fold in the flour, baking soda, baking powder and salt.
4. Put in the chocolate chips then drop spoonfuls of batter on a baking sheet coated with baking paper.
5. Preheat your oven and bake the cookies at 350F for about fifteen minutes or until a golden-brown colour is achieved.
6. Let the cookies cool in the pan before you serve.

Nutritional Content of One Serving:
Calories: 102 | Fat: 5.5g | Protein: 2.1g | Carbohydrates: 11.5g

Peanut Butter Cinnamon Cookies

Total Time Taken: 1 hour
Yield: 20 Servings
Ingredients:

- ¼ cup almond milk
- ½ cup white sugar
- ½ teaspoon baking soda
- ½ teaspoon salt

- 1 ½ cups smooth peanut butter
- 1 cup all-purpose flour
- 1 teaspoon cinnamon powder
- 2 eggs

Directions:

1. Mix the peanut butter, eggs and sugar in a container until creamy.
2. Put in the flour, salt, cinnamon and baking soda and stir for a few seconds to mix.
3. Drop spoonfuls of batter on baking trays covered with parchment paper and preheat your oven and bake the cookies at 350F for about fifteen minutes or until aromatic and crunchy on the edges. These cookies taste best chilled

Nutritional Content of One Serving:

Calories: 168 | Fat: 11.0g | Protein: 6.1g | Carbohydrates: 13.7g

Peanut Butter Cups Cookies

Total Time Taken: 1 ¼ hours

Yield: 25 Servings

Ingredients:

- ¼ cup smooth peanut butter
- ¼ teaspoon salt
- ½ cup butter, softened
- ½ teaspoon baking soda
- ¾ cup light brown sugar
- 1 ½ cups all-purpose flour
- 1 cup peanut butter, chopped
- 1 egg
- 1 teaspoon vanilla extract
- 2 tablespoons golden syrup

Directions:

1. Mix the butter and smooth peanut butter in a container until smooth and creamy.
2. Put in the sugar and golden syrup then mix in the egg and vanilla extract.
3. Put in the flour, baking soda and salt then fold in the peanut butter cups.
4. Drop spoonfuls of batter on a baking tray covered with parchment paper.
5. Preheat your oven and bake the cookies at 350F for about fifteen minutes or until a golden-brown colour is achieved on the edges.
6. *These cookies taste best chilled.*

Nutritional Content of One Serving:

Calories: 160 | Fat: 10.4g | Protein: 4.3g | Carbohydrates: 13.8g

Peanut Butter Nutella Cookies

Total Time Taken: 1 ¼ hours

Yield: 20 Servings

Ingredients:

- ¼ cup butter, softened
- ¼ teaspoon salt
- ½ cup dark brown sugar
- ½ cup Nutella
- ½ cup peanut butter, softened
- ½ teaspoon baking powder
- ½ teaspoon baking soda
- 1 ½ cups all-purpose flour
- 1 egg
- 1 teaspoon vanilla extract

Directions:

1. Mix the butter, peanut butter and sugar in a container until creamy and fluffy.
2. Put in the egg and vanilla and stir thoroughly until blended.
3. Fold in the flour, baking soda, baking powder and salt.
4. Put in the Nutella and swirl it into the batter.
5. Drop spoonfuls of batter on a baking sheet coated with baking paper.
6. Preheat your oven and bake the cookies at 350F for fifteen minutes or until a golden-brown colour is achieved on the edges.
7. *These cookies taste best chilled.*

Nutritional Content of One Serving:

Calories: 120 | Fat: 6.5g | Protein: 3.0g | Carbohydrates: 13.2g

Peanut Butter Oatmeal Cookies

Total Time Taken: 1 ½ hours

Yield: 30 Servings

Ingredients:

- ¼ cup butter, softened
- ¼ cup heavy cream
- ¼ teaspoon salt
- ½ cup light brown sugar
- ½ cup smooth peanut butter
- ½ cup white sugar
- ½ teaspoon baking soda
- 1 cup all-purpose flour
- 1 egg
- 1 teaspoon vanilla extract
- 2 cups rolled oats

Directions:

1. Mix the peanut butter, butter and sugars in a container until pale and creamy.
2. Put in the egg and vanilla and mix thoroughly.
3. Put in the cream as well then fold in the flour, oats, baking soda and salt.
4. Drop spoonfuls of batter on a baking tray coated with baking paper.
5. Preheat your oven and bake the cookies at 350F for about fifteen minutes or until the cookies turn golden-brown on the edges.
6. *These cookies taste best chilled.*

Nutritional Content of One Serving:

Calories: 102 | Fat: 4.6g | Protein: 2.5g | Carbohydrates: 13.5g

Peanut Butter Pretzel Cookies

Total Time Taken: 1 ¼ hours
Yield: 30 Servings
Ingredients:

- ¼ teaspoon salt
- ½ cup smooth peanut butter
- ½ teaspoon baking soda
- ¾ cup butter, softened
- 1 cup crushed pretzels
- 1 cup light brown sugar
- 1 egg
- 1 teaspoon vanilla extract
- 2 cups all-purpose flour

Directions:

1. Mix the butter, peanut butter and sugar in a container until creamy and fluffy.
2. Put in the egg and vanilla and mix thoroughly.
3. Fold in the flour, salt and baking soda then put in the pretzels.
4. Drop spoonfuls of batter on a baking tray coated with baking paper.
5. Pre-heat the oven and bake at 350F for about twenty minutes or until a golden-brown colour is achieved on the edges.
6. *These cookies taste best chilled.*

Nutritional Content of One Serving:
Calories: 121 | Fat: 7.0g | Protein: 2.2g | Carbohydrates: 12.7g

Peanut Butter Shortbread Cookies

Total Time Taken: 2 hours
Yield: 25 Servings
Ingredients:

- ½ cup butter, softened
- ½ cup powdered sugar
- ½ cup smooth peanut butter
- ½ teaspoon baking powder
- ½ teaspoon salt
- 1 ¾ cups all-purpose flour
- 1 egg
- 1 tablespoon cocoa powder
- 1 teaspoon vanilla extract

Directions:

1. Mix the peanut butter, butter, sugar and vanilla in a container until creamy and fluffy.
2. Stir in the egg and mix thoroughly then put in the cocoa powder, flour, salt and baking powder.
3. Cover the dough with plastic wrap and store in the refrigerator for about half an hour.
4. Transfer the dough to a floured working surface and roll it into a slim sheet.
5. Cut into small cookies using a cookie cutter of your choice.
6. Put the cookies in a baking sheet coated with baking paper.
7. Pre-heat the oven and bake at 350F for about fifteen minutes until it is aromatic and appears golden.
8. *These cookies taste best chilled.*

Nutritional Content of One Serving:
Calories: 108 | Fat: 6.6g | Protein: 2.5g | Carbohydrates: 10.3g

Pecan Butter Cookies

Total Time Taken: 1 ¼ hours
Yield: 20 Servings
Ingredients:

- ½ cup pecan butter, softened
- 1 egg
- 1 teaspoon vanilla extract
- 1 cup all-purpose flour
- 1 cup ground pecans
- ¼ teaspoon salt
- ½ teaspoon baking soda
- 1 cup pecans, chopped
- 1/3 cup dark brown sugar

Directions:

1. Mix the butter, sugar, egg and vanilla in a container.
2. Put in the flour, salt, baking soda and ground pecans. Fold in the chopped pecans then drop spoonfuls of batter on a baking tray coated with baking paper.
3. Pre-heat the oven and bake at 350F for about fifteen minutes or until it is aromatic and appears golden-brown on the edges.
4. Serve Chilled and store them in an airtight container.

Nutritional Content of One Serving:
Calories: 86 | Fat: 5.9g | Protein: 1.1g | Carbohydrates: 7.4g

Pecan Cream Cheese Cookies

Total Time Taken: 2 hours
Yield: 40 Servings
Ingredients:

- 1 cup cream cheese
- 1 cup white sugar
- 1 teaspoon vanilla extract
- 1 egg
- 3 cups all-purpose flour
- 1 ½ cups ground pecans
- ¼ teaspoon salt
- 1 teaspoon baking powder
- 2/3 cup butter, softened

Directions:

1. Mix the cream cheese, butter, sugar and vanilla and mix thoroughly. Put in the egg and mix thoroughly.
2. Fold in the remaining ingredients then transfer the dough on plastic wrap and roll it into a log. Wrap tightly and place in the freezer for an hour.
3. Remove the dough from the freezer and cut into thin cookies.
4. Place them on a baking tray coated with baking paper and preheat your oven and bake at 350F for about fifteen minutes or until mildly golden-brown on the edges.
5. *These cookies taste best chilled.*

Nutritional Content of One Serving:
Calories: 105 | Fat: 5.5g | Protein: 1.6g | Carbohydrates: 12.4g

Pecan Marshmallow Cookies

Total Time Taken: 1 ½ hours
Yield: 30 Servings
Ingredients:

- ¼ teaspoon salt
- 1 cup mini marshmallows
- 1 cup pecans, chopped
- 1 cup white sugar
- 1 egg
- 1 teaspoon baking powder
- 1 teaspoon vanilla extract
- 2 ¼ cups all-purpose flour
- 2/3 cup butter

Directions:

1. Mix the butter and sugar in a container until fluffy and creamy.
2. Stir in the vanilla and egg then put in the flour, salt and baking powder.
3. Fold in the pecans and marshmallows then drop spoonfuls of batter on a baking sheet coated with baking paper.
4. Pre-heat the oven and bake at 350F for about fifteen minutes or until a golden-brown colour is achieved on the edges.
5. *These cookies taste best chilled.*

Nutritional Content of One Serving:
Calories: 104 | Fat: 4.7g | Protein: 1.2g | Carbohydrates: 14.7g

Pecan Studded Cookies

Total Time Taken: 1 hour
Yield: 20 Servings
Ingredients:

- ½ cup butter
- 1 teaspoon lemon juice
- 1 egg
- 1 ½ cups all-purpose flour
- ¼ cup cocoa powder
- ¼ teaspoon salt
- ½ teaspoon baking soda
- ½ cup dark chocolate chips
- 2/3 cup light brown sugar

Directions:

1. Melt the butter in a saucepan until it becomes mildly golden brown.
2. Turn off the heat and mix in the lemon juice and egg, as well as sugar.
3. Put in the rest of the ingredients and mix using a spatula.
4. Drop spoonfuls of batter on a baking tray coated with baking paper.
5. Preheat your oven and bake the cookies at 350F for about fifteen minutes or until mildly golden-brown and crisp on the edges.
6. *These cookies taste best chilled.*

Nutritional Content of One Serving:
Calories: 113 | Fat: 5.9g | Protein: 1.7g | Carbohydrates: 14.5g

Pine Nut Cookies

Total Time Taken: 1 hour
Yield: 20 Servings
Ingredients:

- ¼ teaspoon salt
- ½ cup pine nuts
- ½ cup sugar
- 1 ½ cups almond paste
- 1 egg
- 2 egg whites

Directions:

1. Mix the almond paste, sugar and egg and stir thoroughly until creamy.
2. Whip the egg whites and salt until fluffy then fold the meringue into the almond paste.
3. Drop spoonfuls of mixture on baking trays coated with baking paper.
4. Top with pine nuts and preheat your oven and bake at 350F for about fifteen minutes or until a golden-brown colour is achieved and crisp.
5. *These cookies taste best chilled.*

Nutritional Content of One Serving:
Calories: 125 | Fat: 7.3g | Protein: 2.6g | Carbohydrates: 13.6g

Pink Dotted Sugar Cookies

Total Time Taken: 1 ½ hours
Yield: 20 Servings
Ingredients:

- ¼ teaspoon salt
- ½ cup butter, softened
- ½ cup pink sprinkles
- ½ cup powdered sugar
- 1 egg
- 1 teaspoon baking powder
- 2 cups all-purpose flour

Directions:

1. Mix the butter and sugar in a container until fluffy and creamy.
2. Stir in the egg then fold in the flour, salt and baking powder, as well as sprinkles.
3. Transfer the dough to a floured working surface and roll it into a slim sheet.
4. Cut the cookies using a cookie cutter of your choice then arrange them on a baking sheet coated with baking paper.
5. Preheat your oven and bake the cookies at 350F for about fifteen minutes or until a golden-brown colour is achieved on the edges.
6. *These cookies taste best chilled.*

Nutritional Content of One Serving:

Calories: 119 | Fat: 5.0g | Protein: 1.6g | Carbohydrates: 17.5g

Polenta Cookies

Total Time Taken: 1 ¼ hours

Yield: 30 Servings

Ingredients:

- ¼ cup dark brown sugar
- ½ cup light brown sugar
- ½ teaspoon salt
- 1 ¾ cups all-purpose flour
- 1 cup butter, softened
- 1 cup polenta flour
- 1 egg
- 1 egg yolk
- 1 teaspoon baking powder
- 1 teaspoon vanilla extract

Directions:

1. Mix the flours, salt and baking powder in a container.
2. In a separate container, combine the butter and sugars in a container until fluffy and pale.
3. Put in the egg and egg yolk, as well as the vanilla and mix thoroughly.
4. Stir in the flour then drop spoonfuls of batter on a baking sheet coated with baking paper.
5. Pre-heat the oven and bake at 350F for about fifteen minutes or until a golden-brown colour is achieved on the edges.
6. Serve Chilled or store them in an airtight container.

Nutritional Content of One Serving:

Calories: 101 | Fat: 6.5g | Protein: 1.2g | Carbohydrates: 9.7g

Praline Cookies

Total Time Taken: 1 ¼ hours

Yield: 30 Servings

Ingredients:

- ¼ teaspoon salt
- ½ cup butter, softened
- ½ cup light brown sugar
- ½ cup praline paste
- 1 tablespoon praline liqueur
- 1 teaspoon baking soda
- 1 teaspoon vanilla extract
- 2 cups all-purpose flour
- 2 eggs

Directions:

1. Mix the butter, praline paste and sugar in a container until pale and fluffy.
2. Put in the egg yolks, vanilla and praline liqueur and mix thoroughly.
3. Stir in the flour, salt and baking soda then mix using a spatula.
4. Transfer the dough to a floured working surface and roll it into a slim sheet.
5. Cut into small cookies with a cookie cutter and place them all on a baking tray coated with baking paper.
6. Preheat your oven and bake the cookies at 350F for about fifteen minutes or until a golden-brown colour is achieved on the edges.
7. *These cookies taste best chilled.*

Nutritional Content of One Serving:

Calories: 91 | Fat: 4.6g | Protein: 1.5g | Carbohydrates: 10.9g

Puffed Rice Cookies

Total Time Taken: 1 ¼ hours

Yield: 20 Servings

Ingredients:

- ½ cup butter, softened
- ½ cup light brown sugar
- ½ teaspoon salt
- 1 ½ cup all-purpose flour
- 1 egg
- 1 teaspoon baking powder
- 2 cups puffed rice cereals
- 2 tablespoons golden syrup

Directions:

1. Mix the butter, sugar and golden syrup in a container until fluffy and creamy.
2. Put in the egg and mix thoroughly then fold in the remaining ingredients.
3. Drop spoonfuls of batter on a baking sheet coated with baking paper.
4. Pre-heat the oven and bake at 350F for about fifteen minutes or until a golden-brown colour is achieved on the edges.
5. *These cookies taste best chilled.*

Nutritional Content of One Serving:

Calories: 103 | Fat: 4.9g | Protein: 1.4g | Carbohydrates: 13.6g

Quick Brown Butter Cookies

Total Time Taken: 1 hour

Yield: 20 Servings
Ingredients:
- ¼ teaspoon salt
- ½ cup sliced almonds
- ¾ cup butter
- ¾ cup white sugar
- 1 ½ cups all-purpose flour
- 1 egg
- 1 teaspoon baking powder
- 1 teaspoon vanilla extract

Directions:
1. Put the butter in a saucepan and cook it until melted and mildly golden.
2. Let cool and then move to a container and mix in the rest of the ingredients in the same order they are written in.
3. Drop spoonfuls of batter on a baking tray coated with baking paper.
4. Preheat your oven and bake the cookies at 350F for about fifteen minutes or until a golden-brown colour is achieved.
5. *These cookies taste best chilled.*

Nutritional Content of One Serving:
Calories: 141 | Fat: 8.4g | Protein: 1.8g | Carbohydrates: 15.3g

Rainbow Cookies

Total Time Taken: 1 ¼ hours
Yield: 25 Servings
Ingredients:
- ¼ cup coconut oil, melted
- ¼ teaspoon salt
- ½ cup colourful sprinkles
- ½ cup butter, softened
- 1 ½ cups all-purpose flour
- 1 cup white sugar
- 1 egg
- 1 teaspoon baking powder
- 1 teaspoon vanilla extract

Directions:
1. Mix the butter, coconut oil and sugar in a container until fluffy and pale.
2. Stir in the egg and vanilla and mix thoroughly.
3. Fold in the flour, salt and baking powder then put in the sprinkles.
4. Drop spoonfuls of batter on a baking sheet coated with baking paper.
5. Pre-heat the oven and bake at 350F for about fifteen minutes or until a golden-brown colour is achieved on the edges.
6. *These cookies taste best chilled.*

Nutritional Content of One Serving:
Calories: 118 | Fat: 6.3g | Protein: 1.1g | Carbohydrates: 14.8g

Raspberry Jam Cookies

Total Time Taken: 2 hours
Yield: 20 Servings
Ingredients:
- ¼ teaspoon salt
- ½ cup butter, softened
- ½ cup powdered sugar
- ½ cup seedless raspberry jam
- ½ teaspoon baking powder
- 1 ¼ cups all-purpose flour
- 1 cup almond flour
- 1 egg
- 2 tablespoons whole milk

Directions:
1. Mix the butter and sugar in a container until fluffy and creamy.
2. Stir in the egg and milk and mix thoroughly then fold in the flours, salt and baking powder.
3. Transfer the dough to a floured working surface and roll it into a slim sheet.
4. Cut 40 small cookies.
5. Preheat your oven and bake the cookies at 350F for about fifteen minutes.
6. When finished, chill the cookies and fill them two by two with raspberry jam.
7. *Serve immediately.*

Nutritional Content of One Serving:
Calories: 115 | Fat: 5.7g | Protein: 1.5g | Carbohydrates: 14.9g

Rice Flour Cookies

Total Time Taken: 1 hour
Yield: 20 Servings
Ingredients:
- ½ cup butter, softened
- 1 teaspoon vanilla extract
- 1 egg
- ½ cup all-purpose flour
- ½ cup rice flour
- 1 teaspoon baking powder
- ¼ teaspoon cardamom powder
- ¼ teaspoon salt
- 1/3 cup white sugar

Directions:
1. Mix the butter, sugar and vanilla and stir until fluffy.
2. Put in the egg and mix thoroughly then fold in the remaining ingredients.
3. Drop spoonfuls of batter on a baking sheet coated with baking paper.
4. Preheat your oven and bake the cookies at 350F for about fifteen minutes or until a golden-brown colour is achieved on the edges.
5. *These cookies taste best chilled.*

Nutritional Content of One Serving:

Calories: 83 | Fat: 4.9g | Protein: 0.9g | Carbohydrates: 9.1g

Rocky Road Cookies

Total Time Taken: 1 ¼ hours
Yield: 20 Servings
Ingredients:

- ¼ cup light brown sugar
- ½ cup dried cranberries
- ½ cup glace cherries, halved
- ½ cup mini marshmallows
- ½ cup walnuts, chopped
- 1 cup all-purpose flour
- 1 cup macadamia nuts, chopped
- 1/3 cup butter, softened
- 2 eggs

Directions:

1. Mix the butter and sugar in a container until creamy.
2. Put in the eggs, one at a time, then mix in the flour, followed by the remaining ingredients.
3. Drop spoonfuls of batter on a baking tray coated with baking paper.
4. Preheat your oven and bake the cookies at 350F for about fifteen minutes or until a golden-brown colour is achieved on the edges.
5. *These cookies taste best chilled.*

Nutritional Content of One Serving:
Calories: 139 | Fat: 10.5g | Protein: 2.6g | Carbohydrates: 9.7g

Russian Tea Cookies

Total Time Taken: 1 hour
Yield: 30 Servings
Ingredients:

- ¼ teaspoon salt
- ½ cup powdered sugar
- 1 cup butter, softened
- 1 cup ground walnuts
- 1 cup powdered sugar
- 1 egg
- 1 teaspoon baking powder
- 1 teaspoon vanilla extract
- 2 cups all-purpose flour

Directions:

1. Mix the butter and sugar in a container until creamy and pale.
2. Put in the egg and vanilla and mix thoroughly then mix in the flour, walnuts, salt and baking powder.
3. Make small balls of dough and place them on a baking tray coated with baking paper.
4. Transfer the baked cookies in a container and dust them with plenty of powdered sugar.
5. *These cookies taste best chilled.*

Nutritional Content of One Serving:
Calories: 136 | Fat: 8.8g | Protein: 2.1g | Carbohydrates: 12.9g

Salted Chocolate Cookies

Total Time Taken: 1 ½ hours
Yield: 30 Servings
Ingredients:

- ¼ cup cocoa powder
- ½ cup butter
- 1 ½ cups all-purpose flour
- 1 cup light brown sugar
- 1 teaspoon baking powder
- 1 teaspoon sea salt
- 2 cups dark chocolate chips
- 2 eggs
- 2 tablespoons coconut oil
- 2 tablespoons dark brown sugar

Directions:

1. Mix the chocolate and butter in a heatproof container over a hot water bath and melt them together until the desired smoothness is achieved.
2. Put in the coconut oil and mix thoroughly then mix in the sugars and eggs. Stir thoroughly to mix.
3. Fold in the remaining ingredients then drop spoonfuls of batter on a baking sheet coated with baking paper.
4. Preheat your oven and bake the cookies at 350F for fifteen minutes.
5. *These cookies taste best chilled.*

Nutritional Content of One Serving:
Calories: 122 | Fat: 6.5g | Protein: 1.7g | Carbohydrates: 15.9g

Soft Baked Chocolate Cookies

Total Time Taken: 1 ½ hours
Yield: 30 Servings
Ingredients:

- ¼ cup light corn syrup
- ½ cup butter, softened
- ½ teaspoon baking soda
- ½ teaspoon salt
- 1 ¼ cups chocolate chips
- 1 cup dark brown sugar
- 1 teaspoon vanilla extract
- 2 ½ cups all-purpose flour
- 2 eggs

Directions:

1. Mix the butter and sugar in a container until pale and creamy.
2. Put in the corn syrup, eggs and vanilla and mix thoroughly.
3. Fold in the flour, salt and baking soda then put in the chocolate chips and mix thoroughly.
4. Drop spoonfuls of batter on baking trays coated with baking paper and preheat your oven and

bake the cookies at 350F for about fifteen minutes or until a golden-brown colour is achieved and crisp on the edges.

5. *These cookies taste best chilled.*

Nutritional Content of One Serving:

Calories: 133 | Fat: 5.5g | Protein: 2.0g | Carbohydrates: 18.9g

Soft Chocolate Chip Cookies

Total Time Taken: 1 ¼ hours

Yield: 20 Servings

Ingredients:

- ½ cup butter, softened
- ½ teaspoon salt
- 1 cup dark chocolate chips
- 1 cup light brown sugar
- 1 teaspoon baking powder
- 2 cups all-purpose flour
- 2 eggs

Directions:

1. Mix the butter and sugar in a container until fluffy and pale.
2. Put in the eggs, one at a time, stirring thoroughly after each addition.
3. Fold in the remaining ingredients then drop spoonfuls of batter on a baking sheet coated with baking paper.
4. Pre-heat the oven and bake at 350F for about fifteen minutes or until a golden-brown colour is achieved on the edges.
5. *These cookies taste best chilled.*

Nutritional Content of One Serving:

Calories: 148 | Fat: 6.8g | Protein: 2.3g | Carbohydrates: 20.8g

Soft Ginger Cookies

Total Time Taken: 1 ¼ hours

Yield: 30 Servings

Ingredients:

- ¼ teaspoon salt
- ¾ cup butter, softened
- 1 cup white sugar
- 1 egg
- 1 teaspoon baking soda
- 1 teaspoon ground ginger
- 1 teaspoon vanilla extract
- 1/2 teaspoon cinnamon powder
- 2 cups all-purpose flour
- 3 tablespoons molasses

Directions:

1. Mix the flour, salt, baking soda and spices in a container.
2. In a separate container, mix the butter and sugar and mix thoroughly. Put in the egg and molasses and stir thoroughly until blended. Stir in the vanilla.
3. Fold in the flour mixture then drop spoonfuls of batter on baking trays coated with baking paper.
4. Preheat your oven and bake the cookies at 350F for about fifteen minutes or until it is aromatic and appears golden brown.
5. *These cookies taste best chilled.*

Nutritional Content of One Serving:

Calories: 105 | Fat: 4.8g | Protein: 1.1g | Carbohydrates: 14.6g

Spiced Apple Cookies

Total Time Taken: 1 ¼ hours

Yield: 20 Servings

Ingredients:

- ¼ teaspoon salt
- ½ cup coconut oil, melted
- ½ cup light brown sugar
- ½ teaspoon cinnamon powder
- 1 ½ cups all-purpose flour
- 1 egg
- 1 teaspoon baking powder
- 2 red apples, cored and diced
- 2 tablespoons water

Directions:

1. Mix the oil, sugar and egg in a container until fluffy and light.
2. Put in the water and mix thoroughly then mix in the flour, salt, baking powder and cinnamon.
3. Put in the apples then drop spoonfuls of batter on a baking tray coated with baking paper.
4. Preheat your oven and bake the cookies at 350F for about fifteen minutes or until it is aromatic and appears golden brown.
5. *These cookies taste best chilled.*

Nutritional Content of One Serving:

Calories: 108 | Fat: 5.8g | Protein: 1.3g | Carbohydrates: 13.4g

Spiced Chocolate Cookies

Total Time Taken: 1 ¼ hours

Yield: 20 Servings

Ingredients:

- ¼ cup cocoa powder
- ¼ teaspoon salt
- ½ cup butter, softened
- ½ cup dark brown sugar
- ½ teaspoon baking powder
- 1 ¼ cups all-purpose flour
- 1 egg
- 1 teaspoon all-spice powder
- 2 tablespoons honey

Directions:

1. Mix the butter, brown sugar and honey in a container until creamy and fluffy.

2. Put in the egg and mix thoroughly then fold in the flour, cocoa powder, salt, baking powder and all-spice powder.
3. Transfer the dough to a floured working surface and roll it into a slim sheet.
4. Cut the dough using a cookie cutter of your choices and move the cookies to a baking sheet coated with baking paper.
5. Pre-heat the oven and bake at 350F for about twelve minutes.
6. *These cookies taste best chilled.*

Nutritional Content of One Serving:

Calories: 95 | Fat: 5.0g | Protein: 1.4g | Carbohydrates: 11.9g

Sugar Covered Cookies

Total Time Taken: 1 ½ hours

Yield: 30 Servings

Ingredients:

- ¼ teaspoon salt
- ½ cup rice flour
- ½ cup white sugar
- ½ teaspoon baking powder
- 1 cup butter, softened
- 1 cup powdered sugar
- 1 egg
- 1 teaspoon vanilla extract
- 2 cups all-purpose flour
- 2 egg yolks

Directions:

1. Mix the butter and sugar in a container until fluffy and pale.
2. Put in the egg and egg yolks, as well as the vanilla and mix thoroughly.
3. Stir in the rice flour, flour, salt and baking powder in a container.
4. Make small balls and place them on baking trays coated with baking paper.
5. Flatten the cookies then preheat you even and bake at350F for about fifteen minutes or until a golden-brown colour is achieved on the edges.
6. Move the cookies to a container and dust them with powdered sugar.
7. *These cookies taste best chilled.*

Nutritional Content of One Serving:

Calories: 128 | Fat: 6.7g | Protein: 1.4g | Carbohydrates: 15.9g

Thin Coconut Cookies

Total Time Taken: 1 hour

Yield: 20 Servings

Ingredients:

- ¼ cup all-purpose flour
- ¼ teaspoon salt
- ½ cup butter, softened
- ½ cup white sugar
- 1 ¾ cups shredded coconut
- 2 egg whites

Directions:

1. Combine all the ingredients in a container until creamy. Put the dough in your refrigerator until firm.
2. Make small balls of dough and place them on baking trays coated with baking paper.
3. Flatten the cookies and preheat you even and bake at350F for about fifteen minutes or until a golden-brown colour is achieved and crisp on the edges.
4. *These cookies taste best chilled.*

Nutritional Content of One Serving:

Calories: 92 | Fat: 7.0g | Protein: 0.8g | Carbohydrates: 7.3g

Toffee Apple Cookies

Total Time Taken: 1 ¼ hours

Yield: 20 Servings

Ingredients:

- ¼ teaspoon salt
- ½ cup almond flour
- ½ cup butter, softened
- ½ cup toffee bits
- ½ teaspoon baking soda
- 1 ½ cups all-purpose flour
- 1 cup light brown sugar
- 2 apples, peeled and cored
- 2 egg yolks

Directions:

1. Mix the butter and sugar in a container until fluffy and pale.
2. Put in the egg yolks and mix thoroughly then mix in the almond flour, flour, baking soda and salt in the container.
3. Put in the eggs and toffee bits then drop spoonfuls of batter on a baking tray coated with baking paper.
4. Preheat your oven and bake the cookies at 350F for about fifteen minutes or until a golden-brown colour is achieved on the edges.
5. *These cookies taste best chilled.*

Nutritional Content of One Serving:

Calories: 129 | Fat: 5.8g | Protein: 2.1g | Carbohydrates: 17.8g

Toffee Chocolate Chip Cookies

Total Time Taken: 1 ¼ hours

Yield: 30 Servings

Ingredients:

- ¼ cup white sugar
- ½ cup dark chocolate chips
- ½ cup light brown sugar
- ½ teaspoon salt
- 1 cup butter, softened

- 1 cup chopped toffee pieces
- 1 teaspoon baking powder
- 2 ½ cups all-purpose flour
- 2 eggs

Directions:

1. Mix the flour, salt and baking powder in a container.
2. In a separate container, mix the butter and sugars and mix thoroughly. Put in the eggs and stir thoroughly until blended.
3. Put in the flour then fold in the toffee pieces and chocolate chips.
4. Drop spoonfuls of batter on a baking sheet coated with baking paper.
5. Preheat your oven and bake the cookies at 350F for about fifteen minutes or until a golden-brown colour is achieved on the edges.
6. *These cookies taste best chilled.*

Nutritional Content of One Serving:

Calories: 129 | Fat: 7.3g | Protein: 1.7g | Carbohydrates: 14.5g

Triple Chocolate Cookies

Total Time Taken: 1 ¼ hours
Yield: 30 Servings
Ingredients:

- ¼ cup cocoa powder
- ¼ teaspoon baking soda
- ¼ teaspoon salt
- ½ cup dark chocolate chips
- ½ cup dark chocolate chips, melted
- 1 ½ teaspoons baking powder
- 1 cup butter, softened
- 1 cup light brown sugar
- 1 teaspoon vanilla extract
- 2 cups all-purpose flour
- 2 eggs
- 2 tablespoons whole milk

Directions:

1. Mix the butter and sugar in a container until fluffy and pale.
2. Put in the melted chocolate, eggs and vanilla, as well as the milk.
3. Fold in the flour, cocoa powder, baking powder, baking soda and salt then put in the chocolate chips.
4. Drop spoonfuls of batter on a baking sheet coated with baking paper.
5. Preheat your oven and bake the cookies at 350F for about fifteen minutes or until the cookies are golden-brown on the edges.
6. *These cookies taste best chilled.*

Nutritional Content of One Serving:

Calories: 129 | Fat: 7.7g | Protein: 1.7g | Carbohydrates: 14.4g

Vanilla Malted Cookies

Total Time Taken: 1 ¼ hours
Yield: 30 Servings
Ingredients:

- ½ cup cream cheese
- ½ cup malted milk powder
- ½ cup white chocolate chips
- ½ teaspoon baking soda
- ½ teaspoon salt
- 1 cup butter, softened
- 1 cup white sugar
- 1 egg
- 1 teaspoon baking powder
- 1 teaspoon vanilla extract
- 2 ½ cups all-purpose flour

Directions:

1. Sift the flour, milk powder, baking powder, baking soda and salt.
2. Mix the butter, cream cheese and sugar in a container until creamy and fluffy.
3. Put in the vanilla and egg and mix thoroughly.
4. Fold in the flour mixture then put in the chocolate chips.
5. Drop spoonfuls of batter on a baking sheet coated with baking paper.
6. Preheat your oven and bake the cookies at 350F for about fifteen minutes or until a golden-brown colour is achieved on the edges.
7. *These cookies taste best chilled.*

Nutritional Content of One Serving:

Calories: 161 | Fat: 8.8g | Protein: 2.1g | Carbohydrates: 19.0g

Vanilla Sugared Cookies

Total Time Taken: 2 hours
Yield: 20 Servings
Ingredients:

- ¼ teaspoon baking powder
- ¼ teaspoon salt
- ½ cup butter, softened
- ½ cup powdered sugar
- 1 egg
- 1 tablespoon vanilla extract
- 2 cups all-purpose flour
- Powdered sugar for coating the cookies

Directions:

1. Mix the butter and sugar in a container until pale and light.
2. Put in the vanilla and egg and mix thoroughly.
3. Stir in the flour, salt and baking powder then transfer the dough on a plastic wrap and roll it into a log.
4. Wrap the dough and place it in the freezer for about half an hour.

5. When finished, cut the log of dough into thin slices.
6. Put the cookies in a baking tray covered with parchment paper and preheat your oven and bake at 350F for about ten minutes or until a golden-brown colour is achieved on the edges.
7. *These cookies taste best chilled.*

Nutritional Content of One Serving:
Calories: 103 | Fat: 5.0g | Protein: 1.6g | Carbohydrates: 12.7g

Walnut Banana Cookies

Total Time Taken: 1 hour
Yield: 20 Servings
Ingredients:

- ¼ cup dark brown sugar
- ½ cup all-purpose flour
- ½ cup butter, softened
- ½ cup dark chocolate chips
- ½ cup walnuts, chopped
- ½ cup white sugar
- ½ teaspoon baking powder
- ½ teaspoon salt
- 1 banana, mashed
- 1 cup whole wheat flour
- 1 egg
- 1 teaspoon vanilla extract

Directions:

1. Mix the butter and sugars in a container until fluffy and pale.
2. Put in the egg, vanilla and banana and mix thoroughly.
3. Stir in the flours, salt and baking powder then fold in the chocolate chips and walnuts.
4. Drop spoonfuls of batter on a baking tray covered with parchment paper and preheat your oven and bake at 350F for about thirteen minutes or until a golden-brown colour is achieved and crisp on the edges.
5. *The cookies are best served chilled.*

Nutritional Content of One Serving:
Calories: 143 | Fat: 7.6g | Protein: 2.3g | Carbohydrates: 17.7g

Walnut Crescent Cookies

Total Time Taken: 1 ¼ hours
Yield: 20 Servings
Ingredients:

- 1 teaspoon vanilla extract
- ½ teaspoon almond extract
- 1 egg
- 1 cup all-purpose flour
- 1 ½ cups ground walnuts
- ½ teaspoon salt
- ½ teaspoon baking powder
- 2/3 cup butter, softened
- 2/3 cup white sugar

Directions:

1. Mix the butter, sugar, vanilla and almond extract in a container until fluffy and creamy.
2. Put in the egg and mix thoroughly then fold in the flour, walnuts, salt and baking powder.
3. Take small pieces of dough and shape them into small logs.
4. Place them on a baking tray coated with baking paper and preheat your oven and bake at 350F for about fifteen minutes or until a golden-brown colour is achieved on the edges.
5. *These cookies taste best chilled.*

Nutritional Content of One Serving:
Calories: 164 | Fat: 11.9g | Protein: 3.2g | Carbohydrates: 12.5g

White Chocolate Chunk Cookies

Total Time Taken: 1 ¼ hours
Yield: 30 Servings
Ingredients:

- ¼ cup white sugar
- ½ cup butter, softened
- ½ cup cocoa powder
- ½ teaspoon salt
- 1 cup light brown sugar
- 1 teaspoon baking soda
- 1 teaspoon vanilla extract
- 2 cups all-purpose flour
- 2 eggs
- 4 oz. white chocolate, chopped

Directions:

1. Mix the butter and sugars in a container until fluffy and pale.
2. Put in the vanilla and eggs and mix thoroughly.
3. Fold in the flour, cocoa powder, salt and baking soda.
4. Put in the white chocolate chips then drop spoonfuls of batter on baking trays coated with baking paper.
5. Preheat your oven and bake the cookies at 350F for about fifteen minutes or until risen.
6. *These cookies taste best chilled.*

Nutritional Content of One Serving:
Calories: 110 | Fat: 4.8g | Protein: 1.8g | Carbohydrates: 15.8g

White Chocolate Cranberry Cookies

Total Time Taken: 1 ¼ hours
Yield: 30 Servings
Ingredients:

- ¼ cup coconut oil, melted
- ¼ teaspoon cinnamon powder
- ¼ teaspoon salt
- ½ cup butter, softened

- ½ cup dried cranberries
- ½ cup light brown sugar
- ½ cup white chocolate chips
- 1 ½ cups all-purpose flour
- 1 egg
- 1 tablespoon brandy
- 1 teaspoon baking powder

Directions:

1. Mix the butter, coconut oil and sugar in a container until fluffy and pale.
2. Put in the egg and brandy and mix thoroughly.
3. Fold in the remaining ingredients and mix using a spatula.
4. Drop spoonfuls of batter on a baking tray coated with baking paper.
5. Preheat your oven and bake the cookies at 350F for about fifteen minutes or until a golden-brown colour is achieved on the edges.
6. *These cookies taste best chilled.*

Nutritional Content of One Serving:

Calories: 95 | Fat: 6.0g | Protein: 1.0g | Carbohydrates: 9.1g

White Chocolate Pistachio Cookies

Total Time Taken: 1 ¼ hours

Yield: 40 Servings

Ingredients:

- ¼ cup whole milk
- ½ cup light brown sugar
- ½ cup white chocolate chips
- ½ teaspoon baking powder
- ½ teaspoon salt
- 1 cup butter, softened
- 1 cup pistachio, chopped
- 1 cup white sugar
- 1 teaspoon baking soda
- 1 teaspoon vanilla extract
- 2 ½ cups all-purpose flour
- 2 eggs

Directions:

1. Mix the butter and sugars in a container until fluffy and pale.
2. Put in the eggs and mix thoroughly then mix in the vanilla.
3. Put in the rest of the ingredients and mix using a spatula.
4. Drop spoonfuls of batter on baking trays coated with baking paper.
5. Preheat your oven and bake the cookies at 350F for about fifteen minutes or until a golden-brown colour is achieved on the edges.
6. *These cookies taste best chilled.*

Nutritional Content of One Serving:

Calories: 119 | Fat: 6.3g | Protein: 1.6g | Carbohydrates: 14.5g

BONUS: CAKE RECIPES

Cakes hardly need an explanation. Just remember to sift the flour before using in a recipe as it aerates the flour before it is added to the batter. Also, the toothpick is one of the most popular methods to tell if a cake is cooked. Basically you insert a toothpick into the center of the cake, and if the toothpick comes out dry, your cake is done! All righty then, let us jump straight into the recipes!

All Butter Cake

Total Time Taken: 1 ½ hours
Yield: 14 Servings
Ingredients:
Cake:

- ¼ teaspoon salt
- ½ cup whole milk
- 1 cup butter, softened
- 1 cup white sugar
- 1 teaspoon vanilla extract
- 2 cups all-purpose flour
- 2 teaspoons baking powder
- 4 eggs

Frosting:

- 1 cup butter, softened
- 1 teaspoon vanilla extract
- 2 cups powdered sugar

Directions:

1. To prepare the cake, combine the butter, sugar and vanilla in a container until fluffy and creamy.
2. Put in the eggs, one at a time then mix in the milk.
3. Fold in the flour, baking powder and salt then spoon the batter in a 9-inch round cake pan coated with baking paper.
4. Pre-heat the oven and bake at 350F for about forty minutes.
5. Let the cake cool in the pan then cut it in half along the length.
6. For the frosting, combine the butter, sugar and vanilla in a container until fluffy and pale.
7. Use half of the buttercream to fill the cake and the half that is left over to frost the cake.
8. *Serve the cake fresh or chilled.*

Nutritional Content of One Serving:
Calories: 443 | Fat: 28.0g | Protein: 4.0g | Carbohydrates: 45.9g

Almond Apple Cake

Total Time Taken: 1 ¼ hours
Yield: 10 Servings
Ingredients:

- ¼ teaspoon salt
- ½ cup whole milk
- ¾ cup all-purpose flour
- ¾ cup butter, softened
- 1 cup almond flour
- 1 cup white sugar
- 1 teaspoon baking powder
- 1 teaspoon vanilla extract
- 2 red apples, cored and diced
- 3 eggs

Directions:

1. Mix the butter with sugar in a container until creamy.
2. Put in the vanilla and eggs and mix thoroughly then fold in the almond flour, flour, salt and baking powder.
3. Put in the milk and stir lightly then fold in the apples.
4. Spoon the batter in a 8-inch round cake pan coated with baking paper and preheat your oven and bake at 350F for forty minutes or until it rises significantly and seems golden.
5. Let the cake cool in the pan before you serve.

Nutritional Content of One Serving:
Calories: 294 | Fat: 17.1g | Protein: 3.9g | Carbohydrates: 33.7g

Almond Butter Banana Cake

Total Time Taken: 1 ¼ hours
Yield: 12 Servings
Ingredients:

- ¼ cup canola oil
- ½ cup shredded coconut
- ½ teaspoon ground ginger
- ½ teaspoon salt
- 1 ½ cups white sugar
- 1 cup almond butter
- 1 teaspoon baking soda
- 1 teaspoon cinnamon powder
- 1 teaspoon vanilla extract
- 2 bananas, mashed
- 2 cups all-purpose flour
- 3 eggs

Directions:

1. Sift the flour, baking soda, salt, cinnamon and ginger. Combine it with the shredded coconut.
2. Mix the almond butter and sugar in a container until creamy.
3. Stir in the eggs, one at a time, then put in the vanilla, bananas and canola oil. Stir thoroughly to mix.
4. Fold in the flour mixture then pour the batter in a 9-inch round cake pan coated with baking paper.

5. Pre-heat the oven and bake at 350F for about forty-five minutes or until it rises significantly and starts to appear golden-brown.
6. Let the cake cool in the pan before you serve.

Nutritional Content of One Serving:
Calories: 388 | Fat: 18.8g | Protein: 8.3g | Carbohydrates: 49.8g

Almond Date Cake

Total Time Taken: 1 hour
Yield: 8 Servings
Ingredients:
2 eggs

- ¼ cup cocoa powder
- ¼ cup rice flour
- ¼ teaspoon salt
- ½ cup white sugar
- ½ lemon, zested and juiced
- 1 ½ cups almond flour
- 1 cup dates, pitted
- 1 teaspoon baking soda
- 4 egg whites

Directions:
1. Mix the eggs, egg whites, lemon zest, lemon juice, sugar and dates in a food processor.
2. Put in the almond flour, rice flour, cocoa powder, baking soda and salt and stir lightly using a spatula.
3. Pour the batter in a 8-inch round cake pan coated with baking paper.
4. Pre-heat the oven and bake at 350F for around forty minutes.
5. Let the cake cool in the pan before you serve.

Nutritional Content of One Serving:
Calories: 188 | Fat: 4.3g | Protein: 5.6g | Carbohydrates: 35.9g

Almond Fig Cake

Total Time Taken: 1 ¼ hours
Yield: 10 Servings
Ingredients:

- 2 eggs
- 4 egg whites
- 1 cup white sugar
- ½ cup butter, melted
- 1 cup all-purpose flour
- 1 teaspoon baking powder
- ¼ teaspoon salt
- 1 cup ground almonds
- 6 figs, sliced

Directions:
1. Mix the eggs, egg whites and sugar in a container until creamy and volume increases to twice what it was.
2. Put in the melted butter, progressively, then fold in the flour, baking powder, salt and almonds.
3. Pour the batter in a 8-inch round cake pan coated with baking paper.
4. Top with figs and preheat your oven and bake at 350F for around forty minutes or until it rises significantly and starts to appear golden-brown.
5. Let the cake cool in the pan and serve, sliced.

Nutritional Content of One Serving:
Calories: 305 | Fat: 15.1g | Protein: 6.3g | Carbohydrates: 39.3g

Almond Honey Cake

Total Time Taken: 1 ¼ hours
Yield: 10 Servings
Ingredients:

- ¼ cup light brown sugar
- ¼ teaspoon cinnamon powder
- ¼ teaspoon salt
- ½ cup ground almonds
- ½ cup honey
- ½ cup sliced almonds
- ¾ cup butter, softened
- 1 ½ cups all-purpose flour
- 1 teaspoon baking powder
- 3 eggs

Directions:
1. Mix the butter, honey and sugar in a container until creamy and pale.
2. Put in the eggs and mix thoroughly.
3. Fold in the flour, almonds, baking powder, salt and cinnamon powder.
4. Spoon the batter in a loaf cake pan coated with baking paper.
5. Top with sliced almonds and preheat your oven and bake at 350F for forty minutes or until a toothpick inserted into the center of the cake comes out clean.
6. The cake tastes best chilled.

Nutritional Content of One Serving:
Calories: 330 | Fat: 20.1g | Protein: 5.8g | Carbohydrates: 34.2g

Almond Strawberry Cake

Total Time Taken: 1 ¼ hours
Yield: 8 Servings
Ingredients:

- ½ cup butter, softened
- ½ cup white sugar
- ½ cup whole milk
- ½ teaspoon salt
- 1 cup all-purpose flour
- 1 cup fresh strawberries, sliced
- 1 cup ground almonds
- 1 teaspoon baking soda

- 1 teaspoon vanilla extract
- 2 eggs

Directions:

1. Mix the butter and sugar in a container until creamy. Stir in the eggs, one at a time, then put in the milk and vanilla.
2. Fold in the flour, almonds, baking soda and salt and stir lightly.
3. Fold in the strawberries then spoon the batter in a round cake pan coated with baking paper.
4. Preheat your oven and bake the cake for about half an hour or until a golden-brown colour is achieved and it rises significantly.
5. Let the cake cool in the pan before you serve.

Nutritional Content of One Serving:

Calories: 306 | Fat: 19.2g | Protein: 6.2g | Carbohydrates: 29.2g

Almond Strawberry Cake

Total Time Taken: 1 ¼ hours
Yield: 10 Servings
Ingredients:

- ½ cup plain yogurt
- 1 cup all-purpose flour
- 1 cup almond flour
- 1 cup butter, softened
- 1 cup white sugar
- 1 teaspoon baking soda
- 1 teaspoon vanilla
- 2 cups fresh strawberries
- 4 eggs

Directions:

1. Mix the butter with sugar and vanilla in a container until creamy.
2. Stir in the eggs, one at a time, then put in the yogurt and mix thoroughly.
3. Fold in the almond flour, all-purpose flour, baking soda and a pinch of salt and stir lightly using a spatula.
4. Pour the batter in a 9-inch round cake pan and top with strawberries.
5. Pre-heat the oven and bake at 350F for about forty-five minutes or until a toothpick comes out clean after being inserted into the center of the cake.
6. The cake tastes best chilled.

Nutritional Content of One Serving:

Calories: 344 | Fat: 21.9g | Protein: 5.2g | Carbohydrates: 33.4g

Almond White Chocolate Cake

Total Time Taken: 1 ½ hours
Yield: 10 Servings
Ingredients:

- ½ cup dried cranberries
- ½ cup sliced almonds
- ½ cup sour cream
- ½ teaspoon salt
- 1 ½ teaspoons baking soda
- 1 cup all-purpose flour
- 1 cup butter, softened
- 1 cup ground almonds
- 1 cup light brown sugar
- 1 cup white chocolate chips
- 1 tablespoon orange zest
- 3 eggs

Directions:

1. Mix the butter and sugar in a container until creamy and fluffy.
2. Stir in the eggs, one at a time, then put in the orange zest and sour cream.
3. Fold in the flour, almonds, baking soda and salt then put in the cranberries and chocolate chips.
4. Spoon the batter in a 9-inch round cake pan and top with sliced almonds.
5. Pre-heat the oven and bake at 350F for about forty minutes or until it rises significantly and starts to appear golden-brown.
6. Let the cake cool in the pan and serve, sliced.

Nutritional Content of One Serving:

Calories: 485 | Fat: 34.8g | Protein: 7.5g | Carbohydrates: 38.1g

Amaretto Almond Cake

Total Time Taken: 1 hour
Yield: 8 Servings
Ingredients:

- ¼ cup cocoa powder
- ¼ teaspoon salt
- ½ cup butter, softened
- ½ cup light brown sugar
- 1 ½ cups almond flour
- 1 teaspoon baking powder
- 1 teaspoon lemon zest
- 1 teaspoon orange zest
- 2 tablespoons Amaretto
- 3 eggs

Directions:

1. Mix the butter, sugar, orange zest and lemon zest in a container until fluffy and creamy.
2. Put in the eggs, one at a time, then mix in the almond flour, cocoa, salt and baking powder, preferably using a spatula.
3. Spoon the batter in a 8-inch round cake pan and preheat your oven and bake at 350F for 35 minutes or until a toothpick comes out clean after being inserted into the center of the cake.
4. Immediately after you take it out of the oven, sprinkle it with Amaretto.
5. Serve chilled.

Nutritional Content of One Serving:
Calories: 208 | Fat: 16.1g | Protein: 3.8g | Carbohydrates: 12.0g

Apple and Pear Molasses Cake

Total Time Taken: 1 ¼ hours
Yield: 10 Servings
Ingredients:

- ¼ cup butter, softened
- ½ cup canola oil
- ½ cup light molasses
- ½ cup white sugar
- 1 egg
- ½ cup whole milk
- 1 pear, peeled, cored and diced
- 1 red apple, peeled, cored and diced
- 1 teaspoon baking powder
- 1 teaspoon baking soda
- 1 teaspoon cinnamon powder
- 1 teaspoon grated ginger
- 2 cups all-purpose flour

Directions:

1. Mix the canola oil, butter, molasses and sugar in a container until creamy. Put in the egg, ginger and cinnamon and mix thoroughly then mix in the milk.
2. Fold in the remaining ingredients then spoon the batter in a 9-inch round cake pan covered with parchment paper.
3. Pre-heat the oven and bake at 350F for about forty minutes or until a toothpick comes out clean after being inserted into the center of the cake.
4. Let cool in the pan then cut and serve.

Nutritional Content of One Serving:
Calories: 345 | Fat: 16.7g | Protein: 3.7g | Carbohydrates: 46.9g

Apple Pound Cake

Total Time Taken: 1 ¼ hours
Yield: 10 Servings
Ingredients:

- ¼ teaspoon salt
- ½ cup cream cheese, softened
- ½ teaspoon baking soda
- ½ teaspoon cinnamon powder
- ¾ cup butter, softened
- 1 ½ cups all-purpose flour
- 1 cup white sugar
- 1 teaspoon baking powder
- 1 teaspoon vanilla extract
- 2 granny Smith apples, peeled, cored and diced
- 3 eggs

Directions:

1. Mix the butter, cream cheese and sugar in a container until creamy and fluffy.
2. Stir in the eggs and vanilla and mix thoroughly.
3. Fold in the flour, baking powder, baking soda, salt and cinnamon.
4. Put in the apple dices then spoon the batter in a loaf cake pan coated with baking paper.
5. Pre-heat the oven and bake at 350F for forty minutes or until a toothpick inserted into the center of the cake comes out clean.
6. *The cake tastes best chilled.*

Nutritional Content of One Serving:
Calories: 345 | Fat: 19.4g | Protein: 4.7g | Carbohydrates: 40.0g

Apple Vanilla Loaf Cake

Total Time Taken: 1 ¼ hours
Yield: 10 Servings
Ingredients:

- ¼ teaspoon salt
- ½ cup butter, softened
- ½ cup canola oil
- ½ cup cornstarch
- ½ cup whole milk
- ¾ cup white sugar
- 1 cup all-purpose flour
- 1 tablespoon vanilla extract
- 1 teaspoon baking powder
- 2 red apples, cored and diced
- 3 eggs

Directions:

1. Mix the butter, oil and sugar in a container. Stir thoroughly to mix until creamy.
2. Put in the eggs, one at a time, then mix in the milk and vanilla.
3. Fold in the flour, cornstarch, baking powder and salt, then incorporate the apples.
4. Spoon the batter in a loaf cake pan coated with baking paper.
5. Pre-heat the oven and bake at 350F for around forty minutes or until a toothpick inserted into the center of the cake comes out clean.
6. The cake tastes best chilled.

Nutritional Content of One Serving:
Calories: 353 | Fat: 22.0g | Protein: 3.6g | Carbohydrates: 36.5g

Applesauce Carrot Cake

Total Time Taken: 1 ½ hours
Yield: 12 Servings
Ingredients:

- ¼ cup dark brown sugar
- ½ cup canola oil
- ½ cup shredded coconut
- ½ teaspoon baking powder
- ½ teaspoon salt
- 1 cup applesauce

- 1 cup grated carrots
- 1 cup white sugar
- 1 egg white
- 1 teaspoon baking soda
- 1 teaspoon vanilla extract
- 2 ½ cups all-purpose flour
- 2 apples, peeled, cored and diced
- 3 eggs

Directions:

1. Mix the eggs, egg white, sugars and vanilla in a container until fluffy and pale.
2. Stir in the canola oil and applesauce and mix thoroughly then put in the carrots, coconut and apples, as well as the flour, baking soda, baking powder and salt.
3. Stir slowly until mixed using a spatula just until incorporated.
4. Pour the batter in a 9-inch round cake pan and preheat your oven and bake at 350F for about fifty minutes or until fragrant and a toothpick inserted into the center of the cake comes out clean.
5. Let the cake cool in the pan before you serve.

Nutritional Content of One Serving:

Calories: 307 | Fat: 11.6g | Protein: 4.7g | Carbohydrates: 47.6g

Apricot Cake

Total Time Taken: 1 hour

Yield: 10 Servings

Ingredients:

6 eggs

- ½ cup canola oil
- ½ cup sour cream
- ½ teaspoon salt
- 1 ½ teaspoons baking powder
- 1 cup white sugar
- 1 tablespoon lemon zest
- 1 teaspoon vanilla extract
- 2 cups all-purpose flour
- 6 apricots, halved and sliced

Directions:

1. Mix the eggs with sugar, vanilla and lemon zest in a container until fluffy and creamy.
2. Put in the canola oil and sour cream and mix thoroughly.
3. Fold in the remaining ingredients then pour the batter in a 9-inch round cake pan coated with baking paper.
4. Pre-heat the oven and bake at 350F for about forty minutes or until a toothpick inserted in the center comes out clean.
5. Let the cake cool in the pan before you serve.

Nutritional Content of One Serving:

Calories: 337 | Fat: 16.3g | Protein: 6.5g | Carbohydrates: 42.6g

Apricot Yogurt Loaf Cake

Total Time Taken: 1 ¼ hours

Yield: 10 Servings

Ingredients:

- ¼ cup sliced almonds
- ¼ teaspoon salt
- ½ cup butter, softened
- ¾ cup white sugar
- 1 ¼ cups all-purpose flour
- 1 cup plain yogurt
- 1 teaspoon baking powder
- 1 teaspoon vanilla extract
- 2 eggs
- 4 apricots, pitted and sliced

Directions:

1. Mix the butter and sugar in a container until fluffy and pale. Stir in the eggs, one at a time, then put in the yogurt and vanilla and mix thoroughly.
2. Fold in the flour, baking powder and salt.
3. Spoon the batter in a loaf cake pan coated with baking paper.
4. Top with apricots and drizzle with sliced almonds.
5. Pre-heat the oven and bake at 350F for around forty minutes or until it rises significantly and starts to appear golden-brown.
6. Let the cake cool in the pan before you serve.

Nutritional Content of One Serving:

Calories: 247 | Fat: 11.8g | Protein: 4.9g | Carbohydrates: 31.1g

Banana Bundt Cake With Peanut Butter Frosting

Total Time Taken: 1 ¼ hours

Yield: 12 Servings

Ingredients:

Cake:

- ½ teaspoon salt
- 1 cup buttermilk
- 1 cup canola oil
- 1 cup white sugar
- 1 teaspoon vanilla extract
- 2 cups all-purpose flour
- 2 eggs
- 2 ripe bananas, mashed
- 2 teaspoons baking powder

Frosting:

- ½ cup cream cheese
- ½ cup peanut butter, softened
- ½ cup powdered sugar

Directions:

1. To prepare the cake, combine the oil and sugar in a container then mix in the eggs and vanilla. Stir thoroughly to mix then put in the buttermilk and bananas.
2. Fold in the flour, baking powder and salt then spoon the batter in a greased Bundt cake pan.
3. Pre-heat the oven and bake at 350F for about forty minutes or until a toothpick inserted into the center of the cake comes out clean.
4. Move the cake to a platter.
5. For the frosting, combine the ingredients in a container until creamy.
6. Cover the cake with peanut butter frosting and serve fresh.

Nutritional Content of One Serving:
Calories: 453 | Fat: 28.1g | Protein: 7.4g | Carbohydrates: 45.9g

Banana Cake

Total Time Taken: 55 minutes
Yield: 8 Servings
Ingredients:

- ¼ cup butter, softened
- ¼ cup whole milk
- ¼ teaspoon salt
- ½ cup dark chocolate chips
- ½ cup white sugar
- 1 ½ cups all-purpose flour
- 1 teaspoon baking soda
- 2 eggs
- 2 ripe bananas, mashed
- 2 tablespoons dark brown sugar

Directions:

1. Sift the flour, baking soda and salt in a container.
2. Combine the butter, sugars and eggs in a container and stir thoroughly for five minutes.
3. Put in the mashed bananas and milk then fold in the flour, followed by the chocolate chips.
4. Spoon the batter in a round cake pan coated with baking paper and preheat your oven and bake at 350F for about half an hour or until a golden-brown colour is achieved and it rises significantly.
5. Let the cake cool in the pan and serve, sliced.

Nutritional Content of One Serving:
Calories: 273 | Fat: 9.4g | Protein: 4.9g | Carbohydrates: 44.8g

Banana Chocolate Chip Cake

Total Time Taken: 1 ¼ hours
Yield: 12 Servings
Ingredients:

- ¼ teaspoon salt
- ½ cup butter, softened
- ½ cup dark chocolate chips
- ½ cup walnuts, chopped
- 1 ¾ cups all-purpose flour
- 1 cup white sugar
- 1 teaspoon baking soda
- 1 teaspoon vanilla extract
- 3 eggs
- 3 ripe bananas, mashed

Directions:

1. Sift the flour, baking soda and salt on a platter.
2. Mix the butter with sugar until creamy and fluffy.
3. Stir in the eggs, one at a time, then put in the vanilla and bananas.
4. Stir thoroughly to mix then fold in the flour, followed by the walnuts and chocolate chips.
5. Spoon the batter in a 9-inch round cake pan covered with parchment paper.
6. Pre-heat the oven and bake at 350F for about forty minutes or until a toothpick inserted into the center of the cake comes out clean.
7. Let the cake cool in the pan and serve, sliced.

Nutritional Content of One Serving:
Calories: 295 | Fat: 13.4g | Protein: 5.2g | Carbohydrates: 41.3g

Banana Mars Bar Cake

Total Time Taken: 1 ¼ hours
Yield: 10 Servings
Ingredients:

- ½ cup butter, softened
- ½ cup light brown sugar
- ½ cup whole milk
- ½ teaspoon salt
- 2 bananas, mashed
- 2 cups all-purpose flour
- 2 eggs
- 2 Mars bars, chopped
- 2 tablespoons maple syrup
- 2 teaspoons baking powder

Directions:

1. Mix the butter, sugar and maple syrup in a container until fluffy and pale.
2. Put in the eggs and mix thoroughly then mix in the mashed bananas and milk.
3. Fold in the remaining ingredients then spoon the batter in a loaf cake pan coated with baking paper.
4. Pre-heat the oven and bake at 350F for about forty minutes or until a golden-brown colour is achieved and it rises significantly.
5. *The cake tastes best chilled.*

Nutritional Content of One Serving:
Calories: 299 | Fat: 13.1g | Protein: 5.3g | Carbohydrates: 41.6g

Banana Peanut Butter Cake

Total Time Taken: 1 hour
Yield: 8 Servings
Ingredients:

- ¼ cup whole milk
- ½ cup smooth peanut butter
- ½ teaspoon salt
- 1 ½ cups all-purpose flour
- 1 teaspoon baking soda
- 1 teaspoon vanilla extract
- 2 eggs
- 2 ripe bananas, mashed
- 2/3 cup white sugar
- 4 tablespoons butter, softened

Directions:

1. Mix the butter with sugar until creamy and smooth.
2. Stir in the eggs one at a time, then mix in the vanilla and bananas, as well as milk.
3. Fold in the flour, baking soda and salt and mix thoroughly.
4. Spoon the batter in a 9pinch round cake pan coated with baking paper and preheat your oven and bake at 350F for about half an hour or until a golden-brown colour is achieved and it rises significantly.
5. Let the cake cool completely before you serve.

Nutritional Content of One Serving:
Calories: 342 | Fat: 15.6g | Protein: 8.5g | Carbohydrates: 45.0g

Beetroot Carrot Cake

Total Time Taken: 1 ½ hours
Yield: 10 Servings
Ingredients:

- ¼ cup maple syrup
- ½ cup grated beetroots
- ½ cup light brown sugar
- 3 eggs
- ½ cup pecans, chopped
- ½ teaspoon ground cardamom
- ½ teaspoon ground ginger
- ½ teaspoon salt
- ¾ cup vegetable oil
- 1 ½ cups all-purpose flour
- 1 teaspoon baking powder
- 1 teaspoon cinnamon powder
- 1 teaspoon vanilla extract
- 2 cups grated carrots

Directions:

1. Mix the flour, salt, baking powder, cinnamon, ginger and cardamom in a container.
2. In a separate container, combine the oil, maple syrup, sugar, eggs and vanilla until fluffy.
3. Stir in the carrots and beetroots, as well as pecans then fold in the flour.
4. Spoon the batter in a 9-inch round cake pan coated with baking paper.
5. Pre-heat the oven and bake at 350F for about forty minutes or until a toothpick inserted into the center of the cake comes out clean.
6. The cake tastes best chilled.

Nutritional Content of One Serving:
Calories: 305 | Fat: 18.9g | Protein: 4.1g | Carbohydrates: 30.4g

Beetroot Chocolate Fudge Cake

Total Time Taken: 1 ¼ hours
Yield: 10 Servings
Ingredients:

- ¼ cup canola oil
- ¼ teaspoon salt
- ½ cup almond flour
- ½ cup cocoa powder
- 1 ½ cups grated beetroot
- 1 cup all-purpose flour
- 1 cup light brown sugar
- 1 teaspoon baking soda
- 2 tablespoons honey
- 3 eggs

Directions:

1. Mix the eggs with sugar until fluffy and pale. Put in the oil and honey and mix thoroughly.
2. Fold in the flour, cocoa powder, baking soda, almond flour and salt.
3. Put in the beetroot and stir lightly using a spatula.
4. Pour the batter in a 9-inch round cake pan coated with baking paper.
5. Pre-heat the oven and bake at 350F for about half an hour.
6. Let the cake cool in the pan before you serve.

Nutritional Content of One Serving:
Calories: 209 | Fat: 8.2g | Protein: 4.5g | Carbohydrates: 32.5g

Berry Lemon Cake

Total Time Taken: 1 ¼ hours
Yield: 10 Servings
Ingredients:

- ½ cup butter, softened
- ½ cup plain yogurt
- ½ teaspoon salt
- 1 ½ teaspoons baking powder
- 1 cup mixed berries
- 1 cup white sugar
- 1 tablespoon lemon zest
- 2 cups all-purpose flour
- 2 tablespoons lemon juice

- 3 eggs

Directions:

1. Mix the butter and sugar in a container until creamy and fluffy.
2. Stir in the eggs, one at a time, then put in the lemon zest and lemon juice, as well as the yogurt.
3. Fold in the flour, baking powder and salt then put in the berries.
4. Pour the batter in a 8-inch round cake pan and preheat your oven and bake at 350F for around forty minutes or until it rises significantly and starts to appear golden-brown.
5. Let the cake cool in the pan before you serve.

Nutritional Content of One Serving:
Calories: 285 | Fat: 11.0g | Protein: 5.2g | Carbohydrates: 42.3g

Berry Meringue Cake

Total Time Taken: 2 ½ hours
Yield: 8 Servings
Ingredients:

- ½ teaspoon salt
- 1 ½ cups fresh berries
- 1 cup heavy cream, whipped
- 1 cup white sugar
- 1 teaspoon vanilla extract
- 2 tablespoons cornstarch
- 4 egg whites

Directions:

1. Mix the egg whites, salt and sugar in a container. Place over a hot water bath and keep over heat until the sugar is melted.
2. Turn off the heat and whip the egg whites until shiny and fluffy.
3. Fold in the cornstarch then spoon the meringue on a baking sheet coated with baking paper, shaping it into 2 rounds.
4. Pre-heat the oven and bake at 250F for about two hours.
5. Fill and cover the cake with whipped cream and fresh berries.
6. Serve immediately.

Nutritional Content of One Serving:
Calories: 178 | Fat: 5.7g | Protein: 2.3g | Carbohydrates: 30.6g

Black Pepper Chocolate Cake

Total Time Taken: 1 ¼ hours
Yield: 16 Servings
Ingredients:

- ½ teaspoon salt
- 1 ½ cups white sugar
- 1 ½ teaspoons baking powder
- 1 cup butter
- 1 cup sour cream
- 1 teaspoon ground black pepper
- 1 teaspoon lemon zest
- 2 cups all-purpose flour
- 4 eggs

Directions:

1. Mix the flour with baking powder and salt in a container.
2. In a separate container, combine the butter and sugar until fluffy and pale.
3. Stir in the black pepper, lemon zest and eggs and mix thoroughly.
4. Put in the sour cream and give it a good mix.
5. Fold in the flour, baking powder and salt then spoon the batter in a 9-inch round cake pan coated with baking paper.
6. Pre-heat the oven and bake at 350F for about forty minutes or until a toothpick inserted into the center of the cake comes out clean.
7. Let the cake cool in the pan before you serve.

Nutritional Content of One Serving:
Calories: 276 | Fat: 15.8g | Protein: 3.6g | Carbohydrates: 31.7g

Blackberry Bundt Cake

Total Time Taken: 1 ¼ hours
Yield: 10 Servings
Ingredients:

- ½ cup butter, softened
- ½ teaspoon ground cardamom
- ½ teaspoon salt
- 1 cup fresh blackberries
- 1 cup white sugar
- 1 cup whole milk
- 1 teaspoon vanilla extract
- 2 cups all-purpose flour
- 2 eggs
- 2 teaspoons baking powder

Directions:

1. Mix the butter with sugar until creamy, at least five minutes.
2. Put in the eggs and mix thoroughly then mix in the milk and vanilla.
3. Fold in the flour, baking powder, salt and cardamom then put in the blackberries.
4. Spoon the batter in a Bundt cake pan lined using butter.
5. Pre-heat the oven and bake at 350F for around forty minutes or until a toothpick inserted in the center comes out clean.
6. Let the cake cool in the pan for about ten minutes then flip it over on a platter.

Nutritional Content of One Serving:
Calories: 283 | Fat: 11.2g | Protein: 4.8g | Carbohydrates: 42.2g

Blood Orange Cornmeal Cake

Total Time Taken: 1 ½ hours
Yield: 12 Servings
Ingredients:

- ½ teaspoon salt
- 1 cup all-purpose flour
- 1 cup butter, softened
- 1 cup cornmeal
- 1 cup fresh blood orange juice
- 1 cup white sugar
- 2 blood oranges, sliced
- 2 tablespoons blood orange zest
- 2 teaspoons baking powder

Directions:

1. Mix the butter, sugar and orange zest in a container until creamy and fluffy.
2. Mix the flour, cornmeal, baking powder and salt.
3. Stir the flour into the butter mixture, alternating it with the orange juice.
4. Position the orange slices at the bottom of a 9-inch round cake pan coated with baking paper.
5. Pour the batter over the orange slices and preheat your oven and bake at 350F for 45 minutes or until a toothpick inserted into the center of the cake comes out clean.
6. When finished, flip the cake upside down on a platter and serve it chilled.

Nutritional Content of One Serving:
Calories: 298 | Fat: 15.9g | Protein: 2.5g | Carbohydrates: 38.8g

Blood Orange Olive Oil Cake

Total Time Taken: 1 ¼ hours
Yield: 12 Servings
Ingredients:

- ½ cup corn meal
- ½ cup light brown sugar
- ½ teaspoon baking soda
- ½ teaspoon salt
- ¾ cup olive oil
- 1 ½ cups all-purpose flour
- 1 ½ cups white sugar
- 1 cup buttermilk
- 1 teaspoon baking powder
- 2 eggs
- 3 blood oranges, sliced

Directions:

1. Position the blood orange slices in a 10-inch baking tray covered with parchment paper and drizzle them with brown sugar.
2. Mix the oil with eggs and sugar in a container until volume increases to twice what it was.
3. Stir in the flour, baking powder, cornmeal, baking soda and salt then put in the buttermilk and stir for a few seconds to mix.
4. Pour the batter over the orange slices and preheat your oven and bake at 350F for around forty minutes or until a golden-brown colour is achieved and it rises significantly.
5. The cake tastes best chilled, turned upside down on a platter.

Nutritional Content of One Serving:
Calories: 342 | Fat: 13.9g | Protein: 4.2g | Carbohydrates: 54.0g

Blueberry Cake

Total Time Taken: 1 hour
Yield: 12 Servings
Ingredients:

- ½ teaspoon salt
- 1 cup butter, softened
- 1 cup buttermilk
- 1 cup fresh blueberries
- 1 cup white sugar
- 1/4 cup light brown sugar
- 2 tablespoons lemon juice
- 2 tablespoons lemon zest
- 2 teaspoons baking powder
- 3 ½ cups all-purpose flour
- 4 eggs

Directions:

1. Mix the butter and sugars in a container until creamy and fluffy.
2. Stir in the eggs, one at a time, then put in the lemon juice, buttermilk and lemon zest.
3. Fold in the flour, baking powder and salt, followed by the fresh blueberries.
4. Spoon the batter in a 10-inch round cake pan coated with baking paper.
5. Pre-heat the oven and bake at 350F for about forty minutes or until the cake is well risen and golden brown.
6. Let the cake cool in the pan and serve, sliced.

Nutritional Content of One Serving:
Calories: 380 | Fat: 17.4g | Protein: 6.6g | Carbohydrates: 50.9g

Blueberry Streusel Cake

Total Time Taken: 1 ¼ hours
Yield: 10 Servings
Ingredients:
Cake:

- ½ cup sour cream
- ½ teaspoon salt
- ¾ cup butter, softened
- 1 ½ cups fresh blueberries
- 1 cup white sugar
- 1 tablespoon lemon zest
- 1 teaspoon baking soda
- 2 cups all-purpose flour

- 2 tablespoons lemon juice
- 4 eggs

Streusel:

- ¼ cup butter, chilled
- ½ cup all-purpose flour
- 1 pinch salt
- 2 tablespoons powdered sugar

Directions:

1. To prepare the cake, combine the butter, sugar, eggs and sour cream in a container for five minutes until creamy.
2. Put in the lemon zest, lemon juice, flour, baking soda and salt and mix using a spatula.
3. Fold in the fruits then spoon the batter in a 9-inch round cake pan.
4. For the streusel, combine all the ingredients in a container until grainy.
5. Spread the streusel over the cake and preheat your oven and bake at 350F for about forty minutes or until a toothpick inserted in the center comes out clean.
6. Let the cake cool in the pan before you serve.

Nutritional Content of One Serving:

Calories: 421 | Fat: 23.0g | Protein: 6.2g | Carbohydrates: 49.4g

Boozy Chocolate Cake

Total Time Taken: 1 ¼ hours

Yield: 14 Servings

Ingredients:

Cake:

- ¼ cup brandy
- ½ cup canola oil
- ½ cup cocoa powder
- ½ cup hot coffee
- ½ teaspoon salt
- 1 cup buttermilk
- 1 teaspoon baking powder
- 1 teaspoon baking soda
- 2 cups all-purpose flour
- 2 eggs

Frosting:

- ¼ cup brandy
- 1 cup heavy cream
- 2 cups dark chocolate chips
- 2 tablespoons butter

Directions:

1. For the cake, combine the flour, cocoa powder, baking soda, baking powder and salt in a container.
2. Put in the rest of the ingredients and mix thoroughly.
3. Pour the batter in a 9-inch round cake pan , preheat your oven and bake at 330F for 50 minutes.
4. When finished, allow the cake to cool in the pan then move to a platter.
5. For the frosting, bring the cream to the boiling point in a saucepan. Turn off the heat and put in the chocolate. Stir thoroughly to mix until melted and smooth.
6. let the frosting cool down then cover the cake with it.
7. *Serve fresh or chilled.*

Nutritional Content of One Serving:

Calories: 281 | Fat: 18.5g | Protein: 5.1g | Carbohydrates: 28.0g

Boozy Raisin Bundt Cake

Total Time Taken: 2 hours

Yield: 12 Servings

Ingredients:

- ½ cup brandy
- ½ cup whole milk
- ½ teaspoon salt
- 1 ½ cups white sugar
- 1 cup apricot jam
- 1 cup butter, softened
- 1 cup buttermilk
- 1 cup golden raisins
- 2 eggs
- 2 teaspoons baking powder
- 3 cups all-purpose flour

Directions:

1. Sift the flour, salt and baking powder.
2. Mix the butter, sugar and jam in a container until creamy and light.
3. Stir in the eggs, one at a time, then begin incorporating the flour mixture, alternating it with the buttermilk and milk.
4. Spoon the batter in a greased Bundt cake pan and preheat your oven and bake at 350F for about fifty minutes or until a toothpick inserted in the center comes out clean.
5. Let the cake cool in the pan before you serve.

Nutritional Content of One Serving:

Calories: 474 | Fat: 17.0g | Protein: 5.9g | Carbohydrates: 77.5g

Brown Butter Walnut Cake

Total Time Taken: 1 ¼ hours

Yield: 12 Servings

Ingredients:

- ½ teaspoon salt
- 1 ½ cups all-purpose flour
- 1 ½ cups white sugar
- 1 cup butter
- 1 cup ground walnuts
- 1 cup sour cream
- 1 cup walnuts, chopped

- 1 teaspoon baking powder
- 1 teaspoon vanilla extract
- 2 eggs

Directions:

1. Place the butter in a saucepan and melt it. Keep on heat until mildly browned and caramelized. Let the butter cool then move it to a container.
2. Put in the sugar and mix thoroughly.
3. Stir in the eggs and mix thoroughly then put in the sour cream and vanilla.
4. Fold in the flour, baking powder, salt and ground walnuts.
5. Spoon the batter in a 9-inch round cake pan and top with chopped walnuts.
6. Pre-heat the oven and bake at 350F for about forty-five minutes or until a toothpick inserted into the center of the cake comes out clean.
7. *The cake tastes best chilled.*

Nutritional Content of One Serving:

Calories: 468 | Fat: 32.5g | Protein: 8.3g | Carbohydrates: 40.1g

Brown Sugar Cake

Total Time Taken: 1 ¼ hours

Yield: 10 Servings

Ingredients:

- ½ cup dark brown sugar
- ½ teaspoon salt
- 1 cup butter, softened
- 1 cup light brown sugar
- 1 teaspoon vanilla extract
- 2 cups all-purpose flour
- 2 teaspoons baking powder
- 4 eggs
- ½ cup milk

Directions:

1. Sift the flour, baking powder and salt in a container.
2. In another container, combine the butter and sugars until creamy and light.
3. Stir in the eggs, one at a time, then put in the vanilla and milk.
4. Fold in the flour then spoon the batter in a 9-inch round cake pan covered with parchment paper.
5. Pre-heat the oven and bake at 350F for forty minutes or until it rises significantly and starts to appear golden-brown.
6. Let the cake cool in the pan and serve, sliced.

Nutritional Content of One Serving:

Calories: 370 | Fat: 20.7g | Protein: 5.4g | Carbohydrates: 41.7g

Brown Sugar Pineapple Bundt Cake

Total Time Taken: 1 ¼ hours

Yield: 12 Servings

Ingredients:

- ½ cup buttermilk
- ½ cup cornstarch
- ½ cup light brown sugar
- ½ teaspoon salt
- ¾ cup butter, softened
- 1 cup white sugar
- 1 tablespoon lemon zest
- 1 teaspoon baking powder
- 1 teaspoon baking soda
- 1 teaspoon vanilla extract
- 2 cups all-purpose flour
- 3 eggs
- 4 pineapple slices, cubed

Directions:

1. Position the pineapple slices at the bottom of a greased Bundt cake pan and drizzle with brown sugar.
2. Sift the flour with cornstarch, baking soda, baking powder and salt.
3. Mix the butter with sugar in a container until light and creamy then mix in the eggs and vanilla, as well as the lemon zest and buttermilk.
4. Fold in the flour then pour the batter over the pineapple.
5. Pre-heat the oven and bake at 350F for about forty minutes or until it rises significantly and starts to appear golden-brown.
6. Let the cake cool in the pan for about ten minutes then flip it over on a platter.

Nutritional Content of One Serving:

Calories: 332 | Fat: 13.0g | Protein: 4.3g | Carbohydrates: 51.5g

Butter Cake

Total Time Taken: 1 hour

Yield: 8 Servings

Ingredients:

- ¼ teaspoon salt
- ½ cup butter, softened
- ½ cup whole milk
- ¾ cup white sugar
- 1 cup all-purpose flour
- 1 teaspoon baking powder
- 1 teaspoon vanilla extract
- 2 eggs

Directions:

1. Mix the butter, sugar and vanilla in a container until fluffy and pale.
2. Stir in the eggs and mix thoroughly.
3. Fold in the flour, baking powder and salt, alternating it with milk. Begin and finish with flour.
4. Spoon the batter in a 6-inch round cake pan coated with baking paper.

5. Pre-heat the oven and bake at 350F for about half an hour or until a golden-brown colour is achieved.
6. Let the cake cool in the pan before you serve.

Nutritional Content of One Serving:
Calories: 256 | Fat: 13.2g | Protein: 3.6g | Carbohydrates: 31.8g

Buttermilk Chocolate Cake

Total Time Taken: 50 minutes
Yield: 8 Servings
Ingredients:

- ½ cup butter, melted
- ½ cup cocoa powder
- ½ teaspoon salt
- 1 ½ cups all-purpose flour
- 1 cup buttermilk
- 1 cup sugar
- 1 teaspoon baking powder
- 1 teaspoon vanilla extract
- 2 eggs

Directions:
1. Mix the dry ingredients in a container and the wet ingredients in a separate container.
2. Pour the wet ingredients over the dry ones and stir for a few seconds to mix.
3. Pour the batter in a 9-inch cake pan coated with baking paper.
4. Pre-heat the oven and bake at 350F for about half an hour.
5. Let cool in the pan and serve, sliced.

Nutritional Content of One Serving:
Calories: 323 | Fat: 13.8g | Protein: 5.9g | Carbohydrates: 47.8g

Buttermilk Chocolate Cake

Total Time Taken: 1 ¼ hours
Yield: 10 Servings
Ingredients:

- ½ cup cocoa powder
- ½ teaspoon salt
- 1 ¼ cups buttermilk
- 1 cup butter, melted
- 1 cup white sugar
- 1 teaspoon vanilla extract
- 2 cups all-purpose flour
- 2 eggs
- 2 teaspoons baking powder

Directions:
1. Mix all the ingredients in a container.
2. Give it a quick stir until incorporated.
3. Pour the batter in a 9-inch round cake pan coated with baking paper.
4. Preheat your oven and bake the cake for about forty minutes or until the cake is well risen and it passes the toothpick test.
5. Let the cake cool in the pan then serve it chilled.

Nutritional Content of One Serving:
Calories: 365 | Fat: 20.4g | Protein: 5.7g | Carbohydrates: 43.5g

Butterscotch Pecan Cake

Total Time Taken: 1 ½ hours
Yield: 10 Servings
Ingredients:

- ¼ cup canola oil
- ¼ cup cocoa powder
- ¼ cup plain yogurt
- ¼ teaspoon salt
- ½ cup butter, softened
- ½ cup caramel sauce
- 1 ½ cups all-purpose flour
- 1 teaspoon baking powder
- 2 cups pecans
- 2 eggs

Directions:
1. Mix the butter, canola oil, eggs and yogurt in a container until fluffy.
2. Put in the flour, salt, baking powder and cocoa and stir lightly using a spatula.
3. Pour the batter in a 9-inch round cake pan and cover with half of the walnuts.
4. Mix the remaining pecans with caramel and set aside for later.
5. Preheat your oven and bake the cake for around forty minutes.
6. Let cool and then top with butterscotch pecans and serve fresh.

Nutritional Content of One Serving:
Calories: 281 | Fat: 18.1g | Protein: 4.4g | Carbohydrates: 27.4g

Butterscotch Sweet Potato Cake

Total Time Taken: 1 ½ hours
Yield: 10 Servings
Ingredients:
Cake:

- ½ cup canola oil
- ½ cup coconut milk
- ½ cup dark brown sugar
- ½ cup white sugar
- ½ teaspoon salt
- 1 cup sweet potato puree
- 1 teaspoon baking powder
- 1 teaspoon baking soda
- 1 teaspoon cinnamon powder
- 2 cups all-purpose flour
- 3 eggs

Butterscotch sauce:

- ¼ cup butter
- ¼ cup heavy cream
- ¼ cup light corn syrup
- ¼ teaspoon salt
- ½ cup dark brown sugar

Directions:

1. To prepare the cake, combine the dry ingredients in a container and the wet ingredients in a separate container.
2. Combine the dry ingredients with the wet ingredients and give it a good mix.
3. Pour the batter in a 10-inch round cake pan coated with baking paper and preheat your oven and bake at 350F for around forty minutes.
4. Let the cake cool in the pan then move to a platter.
5. For the butterscotch sauce, combine all the ingredients in a saucepan and cook for about five to eight minutes until it becomes thick.
6. Let cool and then pour the sauce over each slice of cake before you serve.

Nutritional Content of One Serving:

Calories: 426 | Fat: 21.1g | Protein: 5.1g | Carbohydrates: 56.2g

Buttery Orange Cake

Total Time Taken: 1 hour

Yield: 8 Servings

Ingredients:

- ¼ cup canola oil
- ½ cup butter, softened
- ½ teaspoon salt
- ¾ cup whole milk
- 1 cup white sugar Zest of
- 1 lemon
- 1 lemon Juice of
- 2 cups all-purpose flour
- 2 teaspoons baking powder
- 4 eggs

Directions:

1. Mix the flour with baking powder and salt.
2. Mix the butter and eggs in a container for five minutes until creamy then put in the eggs, one at a time, as well as lemon juice and zest.
3. Fold in the flour mixture, alternating it with milk. Begin with flour and finish with flour.
4. Spoon the batter in a 9-inch round cake pan coated with baking paper.
5. Pre-heat the oven and bake at 350F for around forty minutes or until a golden-brown colour is achieved and it rises significantly.
6. Let the cake cool in the pan and serve, sliced.

Nutritional Content of One Serving:

Calories: 417 | Fat: 21.6g | Protein: 6.9g | Carbohydrates: 50.8g

Buttery Zucchini Cake

Total Time Taken: 1 ½ hours

Yield: 10 Servings

Ingredients:

- ½ cup dark brown sugar
- ½ cup dark chocolate chips
- ½ teaspoon salt
- 1 cup butter, softened
- 1 cup grated zucchinis
- 1 teaspoon baking powder
- 1 teaspoon baking soda
- 1/2 cup white sugar
- 2 cups all-purpose flour
- 4 eggs

Directions:

1. Mix the butter, brown sugar and white sugar in a container until creamy and firm.
2. Stir in the eggs, one at a time, then put in the zucchinis.
3. Fold in the remaining ingredients then pour the batter in a round cake pan coated with baking paper.
4. Preheat your oven and bake the cake for about forty minutes or until a toothpick inserted in the center comes out clean.
5. Let the cake cool in the pan then serve, sliced.

Nutritional Content of One Serving:

Calories: 374 | Fat: 22.0g | Protein: 5.5g | Carbohydrates: 40.9g

Candied Ginger Applesauce Cake

Total Time Taken: 1 ¼ hours

Yield: 10 Servings

Ingredients:

- ¼ cup candied ginger, chopped
- ¼ teaspoon baking soda
- ½ cup butter, room temperature
- ½ cup golden raisins
- ½ teaspoon cinnamon powder
- ½ teaspoon ground star anise
- ½ teaspoon salt
- 1 ¼ cups applesauce
- 1 cup white sugar
- 1 teaspoon vanilla extract
- 2 cups all-purpose flour
- 2 eggs
- 2 tablespoons molasses
- 2 teaspoons baking powder

Directions:

1. Mix the flour, baking powder, baking soda, salt and spices in a container.

2. In a separate container, combine the butter, sugar and molasses until creamy and firm. Put in the eggs, one at a time, then the applesauce and vanilla and mix thoroughly.
3. Fold in the flour mixture then put in the raisins and ginger.
4. Spoon the batter in a 9-inch round cake pan coated with baking paper.
5. Pre-heat the oven and bake at 350F for about forty minutes or until a golden-brown colour is achieved and it rises significantly.
6. Let the cake cool in the pan and serve, sliced.

Nutritional Content of One Serving:
Calories: 310 | Fat: 10.4g | Protein: 4.1g | Carbohydrates: 52.1g

Caramel Apple Cake

Total Time Taken: 1 ½ hours
Yield: 12 Servings
Ingredients:
Cake:

- ½ cup applesauce
- ½ teaspoon cinnamon powder
- ½ teaspoon ground ginger
- ½ teaspoon salt
- 1 ¼ cups white sugar
- 1 cup butter, softened
- 1 teaspoon baking soda
- 2 cups all-purpose flour
- 2 red apples, cored and diced
- 4 eggs

Glaze:

- ¼ teaspoon salt
- ½ cup heavy cream
- 1 cup white sugar

Directions:
1. For the cake, combine the sugar, butter and eggs in a container until creamy.
2. Stir in the applesauce then put in the flour, baking soda, salt and cinnamon, as well as ginger and apples.
3. Spoon the batter in a 9-inch round cake pan coated with baking paper.
4. Pre-heat the oven and bake at 350F for about forty-five minutes.
5. Let the cake cool in the pan then move to a platter.
6. For the glaze, melt the sugar in a heavy saucepan until it sppears amber in colour.
7. Put in the cream and salt and stir until melted and smooth.
8. let the glaze cool in the pan then sprinkle it over the cake.

Nutritional Content of One Serving:
Calories: 411 | Fat: 18.9g | Protein: 4.4g | Carbohydrates: 59.1g

Caramel Banana Cake

Total Time Taken: 1 hour
Yield: 12 Servings
Ingredients:

- ¼ cup dark brown sugar
- ½ cup caramel sauce
- ½ teaspoon ground cardamom
- ½ teaspoon salt
- ¾ cup butter, softened
- 1 cup buttermilk
- 1 cup white sugar
- 1 teaspoon cinnamon powder
- 2 cups all-purpose flour
- 2 ripe bananas, mashed
- 2 teaspoons baking powder
- 4 eggs

Directions:
1. Mix the butter with sugars for five minutes until creamy. Put in the eggs, one at a time, then mix in the bananas.
2. Fold in the flour, spices, baking powder and salt, alternating it with buttermilk.
3. Pour the batter in a 9-inch round cake pan.
4. Sprinkle the batter with caramel sauce and preheat your oven and bake the cake at 350F for about forty-five minutes or until a toothpick inserted in the center comes out clean.
5. Let the cake cool in the pan and serve, sliced.

Nutritional Content of One Serving:
Calories: 334 | Fat: 13.4g | Protein: 5.2g | Carbohydrates: 50.6g

Caramel Pineapple Upside Down Cake

Total Time Taken: 1 ½ hours
Yield: 14 Servings
Ingredients:

- ¼ cup whole milk
- ¼ teaspoon salt
- ½ cup butter, softened
- ½ cup canola oil
- ½ cup cornstarch
- ½ cup light brown sugar
- ½ cup white sugar
- 1 cup all-purpose flour
- 1 cup shredded coconut
- 1 teaspoon baking soda
- 2 tablespoons butter
- 3 eggs
- 6 slices pineapple

Directions:
1. Melt the white sugar in a saucepan until it sppears amber in colour.

2. Sprinkle the melted sugar on the bottom of a 9-inch round cake pan coated with baking paper.
3. Top the caramelized sugar with butter and set aside for later.
4. For the batter, combine the butter, oil and brown sugar until fluffy and creamy.
5. Fold in the eggs and milk then put in the remaining ingredients and mix using a spatula.
6. Spoon the batter over the pineapple slices and preheat your oven and bake at 350F for about forty minutes or until a toothpick inserted in the center comes out clean.
7. Let the cake cool in the pan for about ten minutes then flip it over on a platter.
8. Serve chilled.

Nutritional Content of One Serving:
Calories: 309 | Fat: 19.2g | Protein: 2.9g | Carbohydrates: 33.6g

Caramel Pumpkin Cake

Total Time Taken: 1 ½ hours
Yield: 12 Servings
Ingredients:
Cake:

- ¼ cup white sugar
- ¼ cup whole milk
- ½ cup coconut oil, melted
- 1 cup dark brown sugar
- 1 cup pumpkin puree
- 1 pinch salt
- 1 teaspoon baking powder
- 1 teaspoon baking soda
- 1 teaspoon cinnamon powder
- 1 teaspoon ground ginger
- 2 cups all-purpose flour
- 4 eggs

Caramel frosting:

1. 1 cup butter, softened
2. 2 cups powdered sugar
3. 1 pinch salt
4. ½ cup caramel sauce

Directions:

1. For the cake, combine the flour, baking powder, baking soda, spices and salt in a container.
2. In a separate container, mix the coconut oil, pumpkin puree, eggs, sugars and milk.
3. Pour this mixture over the dry ingredients and mix thoroughly.
4. Pour the batter in 2 circular cake pans coated with baking paper.
5. Preheat your oven and bake the cake at 350F for 35 minutes or until it rises completely and is aromatic.
6. Let the cakes cool in the pans then level them and set aside for later.
7. For the frosting, combine the butter, sugar and salt in a container for about five to seven minutes or until twofold in volume and firm.
8. Stir in the caramel sauce.
9. Use half of the frosting to fill the cake and the half that is left over to garnish the cake.
10. Serve fresh.

Nutritional Content of One Serving:
Calories: 495 | Fat: 26.4g | Protein: 4.8g | Carbohydrates: 63.2g

Caramel Spice Cake

Total Time Taken: 1 ¼ hours
Yield: 8 Servings
Ingredients:
Cake:

- ¼ teaspoon ground nutmeg
- ½ cup butter, softened
- ½ cup sour cream
- ½ teaspoon ground cardamom
- ½ teaspoon ground ginger
- ¾ cup light brown sugar
- 1 1/4 cups all-purpose flour
- 1 teaspoon baking soda
- 1 teaspoon cinnamon powder
- 3 eggs

Glaze:

- ½ cup heavy cream
- ½ teaspoon salt
- 1 cup white sugar

Directions:

1. For the cake, sift the flour, baking soda, spices and salt in a container.
2. In a separate container, combine the butter and sugar until creamy. Stir in the eggs and mix thoroughly then put in the sour cream and mix thoroughly.
3. Fold in the flour mixture then pour the batter in a 9-inch round cake pan covered with parchment paper.
4. Pre-heat the oven and bake at 350F for around forty minutes or until a toothpick inserted in the center comes out clean.
5. Let the cake cool in the pan.
6. For the glaze, melt the sugar in a heavy saucepan until it sppears amber in colour.
7. Stir in the cream and salt and mix thoroughly. Keep over low heat until the desired smoothness is achieved.
8. Let the glaze cool down then sprinkle it over the cake just before you serve.

Nutritional Content of One Serving:
Calories: 400 | Fat: 19.2g | Protein: 4.9g | Carbohydrates: 54.4g

Cardamom Carrot Cake

Total Time Taken: 1 ¼ hours
Yield: 16 Servings
Ingredients:
Cake:

- ¼ cup dark brown sugar
- ½ teaspoon baking powder
- ½ teaspoon salt
- 1 cup crushed pineapple
- 1 cup pecans, chopped
- 1 cup shredded coconut
- 1 cup vegetable oil
- 1 cup white sugar
- 1 teaspoon baking soda
- 1 teaspoon ground cardamom
- 1 teaspoon vanilla extract
- 2 cups all-purpose flour
- 2 cups grated carrots
- 4 eggs

Frosting:

- ½ cup butter, softened
- 1 cup cream cheese
- 1 cup powdered sugar
- 1 teaspoon vanilla extract

Directions:

1. For the cake, sift the flour, baking soda, baking powder, salt and cardamom in a container.
2. In a separate container, combine the eggs and sugars until creamy and fluffy.
3. Put in the vanilla, carrots, pineapple, coconut and pecans and mix thoroughly.
4. Fold in the dry ingredients then pour the batter into a 10-inch round cake pan coated with baking paper.
5. Preheat your oven and bake the cake for about fifty minutes or until it rises completely and is aromatic.
6. For the frosting, combine all the ingredients in a container for minimum five minutes.
7. Frost the chilled cake with the cream cheese buttercream and serve fresh or place in your refrigerator.

Nutritional Content of One Serving:
Calories: 416 | Fat: 28.0g | Protein: 4.6g | Carbohydrates: 38.4g

Chai Spiced Cake

Total Time Taken: 1 ½ hours
Yield: 10 Servings
Ingredients:
Cake:

- ¼ teaspoon ground cloves
- ½ teaspoon ground ginger
- ½ teaspoon salt
- ½ teaspoon turmeric
- 1 ½ cups white sugar
- 1 cup butter, softened
- 1 teaspoon cinnamon powder
- 1 teaspoon vanilla extract
- 2 cups all-purpose flour
- 2 teaspoons baking powder
- 6 eggs

Frosting:

- ¼ cup light brown sugar
- ½ cup butter, softened
- 1 cup cream cheese
- 1 teaspoon grated ginger
- 2 cups powdered sugar

Directions:

1. For the cake, sift the flour with baking powder, salt and spices on a platter.
2. Mix the butter and sugar in a container until pale and thick.
3. Put in the eggs, one at a time, then mix in the dry ingredients, mixing gently using a spatula.
4. Spoon the batter in a 9-inch round cake pan coated with baking paper.
5. For the frosting, combine the cream cheese, butter and brown sugar in a container for minimum five minutes.
6. Put in the rest of the ingredients and mix thoroughly. Cover the cake with buttercream and serve fresh.

Nutritional Content of One Serving:
Calories: 484 | Fat: 27.6g | Protein: 5.7g | Carbohydrates: 55.8g

Chai Spiced Streusel Cake

Total Time Taken: 1 hour
Yield: 10 Servings
Ingredients:
Streusel:

- ¼ cup all-purpose flour
- ¼ cup butter, melted
- ¼ cup light brown sugar
- ½ teaspoon cardamom powder
- ½ teaspoon cinnamon powder
- ½ teaspoon ground cloves
- ½ teaspoon star anise
- 1 cup pecans, chopped

Cake:

- ¼ cup butter, melted
- ¼ cup whole milk
- ½ cup white sugar
- 1 ¼ cups all-purpose flour
- 1 pinch salt
- 1 teaspoon baking powder
- 6 eggs, room temperature

Directions:

1. Mix the eggs, sugar and salt for minimum five minutes until its volume increases to almost three times it was.

2. Put in the milk then fold in the flour and baking powder.
3. Progressively mix in the melted butter then pour the batter in a 9-inch cake pan coated with baking paper.
4. For the streusel, combine all the ingredients in a container and stir thoroughly until grainy.
5. Spread the streusel over the cake and preheat your oven and bake at 350F for about forty minutes or until a golden-brown colour is achieved and fragrant.
6. Let cool in the pan and serve, sliced.

Nutritional Content of One Serving:

Calories: 254 | Fat: 13.3g | Protein: 5.7g | Carbohydrates: 29.0g

Cherry Brownie Cake

Total Time Taken: 1 hour
Yield: 8 Servings
Ingredients:

- ¼ teaspoon salt
- ¾ cup butter
- ¾ cup light brown sugar
- 1 cup all-purpose flour
- 1 cup cherries, pitted
- 1 cup dark chocolate chips
- 1 teaspoon vanilla extract
- 3 eggs

Directions:

1. Mix the butter and chocolate chips in a heatproof container. Place over a hot water bath and melt them until the desired smoothness is achieved.
2. Turn off the heat and mix in the eggs, vanilla and sugar.
3. Fold in the flour and salt then pour the batter in a 8-inch round cake pan coated with baking paper.
4. Top with cherries and preheat your oven and bake at 350F for 20 minutes.
5. *The cake tastes best chilled.*

Nutritional Content of One Serving:

Calories: 367 | Fat: 23.1g | Protein: 4.9g | Carbohydrates: 38.1g

Cherry Chocolate Cake

Total Time Taken: 1 ¼ hours
Yield: 10 Servings
Ingredients:

- ¼ teaspoon salt
- ½ cup butter, melted
- ½ cup milk
- ½ cup pine nuts, ground
- 1 ½ cups all-purpose flour
- 1 cup white sugar
- 1 teaspoon baking powder
- 1 teaspoon vanilla extract
- 2 cups cherries, pitted
- 3 eggs

Directions:

1. Mix the eggs and sugar in a container until volume increases to twice what it was.
2. Stir in the milk then progressively pour in the butter, stirring thoroughly.
3. Put in the vanilla then fold in the flour, baking powder and salt.
4. Put in the ground pine nuts then fold in the cherries.
5. Pour the batter in a 9-inch round cake pan coated with baking paper.
6. Pre-heat the oven and bake at 350F for about forty minutes or until a toothpick inserted into the center of the cake comes out clean.
7. Let the cake cool in the pan before you serve.

Nutritional Content of One Serving:

Calories: 314 | Fat: 15.6g | Protein: 5.1g | Carbohydrates: 40.3g

Cherry Liqueur Soaked Cake

Total Time Taken: 1 ¼ hours
Yield: 8 Servings
Ingredients:

- ¼ cup cherry liqueurs
- ¼ cup dark brown sugar
- ¼ teaspoon salt
- ½ cup all-purpose flour
- ½ cup butter, melted
- ½ cup hot coffee
- ½ cup white sugar
- ½ teaspoon baking powder
- 1 ½ cups dark chocolate chips
- 1 cup almond flour
- 2 eggs

Directions:

1. Mix the coffee and chocolate in a container. Stir until melted and smooth.
2. Stir in the sugars, butter and eggs then fold in the almond flour, all-purpose flour, salt and baking powder.
3. Pour the batter in a 8-inch round cake pan coated with baking paper.
4. Pre-heat the oven and bake at 350F for a little more than half an hour.
5. Let the cake cool down then move to a platter.
6. Brush the cherry liqueur over the cake.
7. *The cake tastes best chilled.*

Nutritional Content of One Serving:

Calories: 343 | Fat: 20.8g | Protein: 4.6g | Carbohydrates: 39.7g

Chestnut Puree Chocolate Cake

Total Time Taken: 1 ¼ hours
Yield: 10 Servings
Ingredients:

- ¼ cup butter
- ¼ teaspoon salt
- ½ cup canola oil
- ½ cup cocoa powder
- ½ cup ground almonds
- 1 cup all-purpose flour
- 1 cup chestnut puree
- 1 cup dark chocolate chips
- 1 cup white sugar
- 1 teaspoon baking powder

Directions:

1. Mix the canola oil, butter and chocolate chips in a heatproof container. Place over heatproof container and melt them together.
2. Turn off the heat and mix in the sugar and chestnut puree.
3. Fold in the cocoa powder, flour, almonds, salt and baking powder.
4. Spoon the batter in a 9-inch round cake pan coated with baking paper.
5. Pre-heat the oven and bake at 350F for around forty minutes or until a toothpick inserted into the center of the cake comes out clean.
6. The cake tastes best chilled.

Nutritional Content of One Serving:
Calories: 354 | Fat: 21.8g | Protein: 3.9g | Carbohydrates: 41.6g

Chia Seed Chocolate Cake

Total Time Taken: 1 ¼ hours
Yield: 10 Servings
Ingredients:

- ¼ cup cocoa powder
- ¼ teaspoon salt
- ½ cup butter
- ½ cup dark chocolate chips
- 1 ½ cups all-purpose flour
- 1 cup canola oil
- 1 cup white sugar
- 1 tablespoon orange zest
- 1 teaspoon baking powder
- 2 tablespoons chia seeds
- 3 eggs

Directions:

1. Melt the chocolate and butter in a container until the desired smoothness is achieved.
2. Turn off the heat and mix in the eggs, orange zest, sugar and canola oil.
3. Fold in the cocoa powder, chia seeds, flour, baking powder and salt then pour the batter in a 9-inch round cake pan coated with baking paper.
4. Pre-heat the oven and bake at 350F for around forty minutes or until a toothpick inserted into the center of the cake comes out clean.
5. *The cake tastes best chilled.*

Nutritional Content of One Serving:
Calories: 470 | Fat: 34.4g | Protein: 4.5g | Carbohydrates: 40.0g

Chocolate Biscuit Cake

Total Time Taken: 3 hours
Yield: 10 Servings
Ingredients:

- ¼ cup cocoa powder
- ¼ cup dried cranberries
- ½ cup butter
- ½ cup dark chocolate chips
- ½ cup golden syrup
- ½ cup milk chocolate chips
- ½ cup pecans, chopped
- 1 cup golden raisins
- 1 cup heavy cream
- 1 cup milk
- 10 oz. digestive biscuits, chopped

Directions:

1. Melt the chocolate chips and butter in a heatproof container over a hot water bath.
2. Mix the cream, milk and cocoa powder and place over low heat. Bring to a boil and cook just until slightly thickened. Turn off the heat and mix in the chocolate mixture.
3. Mix this mixture with the remaining ingredients in a container then transfer in a 8-inch cake pan coated with plastic wrap.
4. Place in your refrigerator to set for about two hours then serve, sliced.

Nutritional Content of One Serving:
Calories: 408 | Fat: 24.0g | Protein: 4.3g | Carbohydrates: 49.1g

Chocolate Bundt Cake

Total Time Taken: 1 ¼ hours
Yield: 10 Servings
Ingredients:

- ½ cup butter, softened
- ½ cup cocoa powder
- ½ cup dark chocolate chips
- ½ teaspoon baking soda
- ½ teaspoon salt
- 1 ½ cups all-purpose flour
- 1 cup white sugar
- 1 teaspoon baking powder
- 1 teaspoon vanilla extract
- 2 tablespoons canola oil
- 3 eggs

Directions:

1. Mix the butter, canola oil and sugar in a container until light and pale.
2. Stir in the eggs and vanilla and mix thoroughly.
3. Fold in the flour, cocoa powder, baking powder, baking soda and salt.
4. Put in the chocolate chips then spoon the batter in a greased Bundt cake pan.
5. Pre-heat the oven and bake at 350F for about forty minutes or until well risen and it passes the toothpick test.
6. Let the cake cool in the pan and serve, sliced.

Nutritional Content of One Serving:
Calories: 308 | Fat: 15.7g | Protein: 4.9g | Carbohydrates: 41.1g

Chocolate Chip Blackberry Cake

Total Time Taken: 1 ¼ hours
Yield: 10 Servings
Ingredients:

- ¼ cup canola oil
- ¼ cup cornstarch
- ¼ teaspoon salt
- ½ cup butter, softened
- ½ cup dark chocolate chips
- ½ cup plain yogurt
- 1 ½ cups all-purpose flour
- 1 cup fresh blackberries
- 1 cup white sugar
- 1 teaspoon baking powder
- 3 eggs

Directions:
1. Mix the butter, oil and sugar in a container until creamy and fluffy.
2. Put in the eggs and yogurt and mix thoroughly.
3. Fold in the flour, cornstarch, baking powder and salt and mix using a spatula.
4. Put in the chocolate chips and blackberries then spoon the batter in a 9-inch round cake pan coated with baking paper.
5. Preheat your oven and bake the cake for about forty minutes or until it rises significantly and starts to appear golden-brown.
6. Let the cake cool in the pan before you serve.

Nutritional Content of One Serving:
Calories: 347 | Fat: 18.0 | Protein: 5.0g | Carbohydrates: 43.8g

Chocolate Chip Bundt Cake

Total Time Taken: 1 ¼ hours
Yield: 12 Servings
Ingredients:

- ½ teaspoon salt
- ¾ cup dark chocolate chips
- 1 cup butter, softened
- 1 cup plain yogurt
- 1 cup white sugar
- 1 teaspoon vanilla extract
- 2 cups all-purpose flour
- 2 teaspoons baking powder
- 3 eggs

Directions:
1. Mix the flour with baking powder and salt.
2. Mix the butter with sugar until creamy. Put in the eggs, one at a time, then mix in the vanilla and mix thoroughly.
3. Put in the yogurt and mix thoroughly then fold in the flour, followed by the chocolate chips.
4. Spoon the batter in a greased Bundt cake pan.
5. Pre-heat the oven and bake at 350F for about forty minutes or until a toothpick inserted in the cake comes out clean.

Nutritional Content of One Serving:
Calories: 341 | Fat: 18.9g | Protein: 5.3g | Carbohydrates: 39.5g

Chocolate Chip Pumpkin Bundt Cake

Total Time Taken: 1 ¼ hours
Yield: 12 Servings
Ingredients:

- ½ teaspoon salt
- 1 ½ cups white sugar
- 1 ½ teaspoons baking powder
- 1 cup butter, softened
- 1 cup dark chocolate chips
- 1 cup pumpkin puree
- 1 teaspoon vanilla extract
- 2 cups all-purpose flour
- 2 eggs
- 2 tablespoons molasses

Directions:
1. Mix the butter, sugar and molasses in a container until creamy and light.
2. Stir in the vanilla and eggs, as well as the pumpkin puree.
3. Fold in the remaining ingredients and stir lightly.
4. Spoon the batter in a greased Bundt cake pan. Pre-heat the oven and bake at 350F for about forty-five minutes or until a toothpick inserted into the center of the cake comes out clean.
5. Let the cake cool in the pan before you serve.

Nutritional Content of One Serving:
Calories: 381 | Fat: 19.0g | Protein: 4.1g | Carbohydrates: 52.1g

Chocolate Coconut Cake

Total Time Taken: 1 ¼ hours
Yield: 10 Servings
Ingredients:

- ¼ cup cocoa powder
- ¼ teaspoon salt
- ½ cup butter
- ¾ cup milk
- 1 ½ cups all-purpose flour
- 1 cup shredded coconut
- 1 cup white sugar
- 1 teaspoon baking powder
- 2 eggs
- 2 tablespoons canola oil

Directions:

1. Mix the butter, oil and sugar in a container until fluffy and creamy.
2. Put in the eggs, one at a time, then mix in the milk.
3. Put in the dry ingredients and stir lightly using a spatula.
4. Spoon the batter in a 8-inch round cake pan coated with baking paper.
5. Pre-heat the oven and bake at 350F for around forty minutes or until a toothpick inserted into the center of the cake comes out clean.
6. *The cake tastes best chilled.*

Nutritional Content of One Serving:
Calories: 305 | Fat: 16.4g | Protein: 4.4g | Carbohydrates: 37.9g

Chocolate Coffee Cake

Total Time Taken: 1 hour
Yield: 12 Servings
Ingredients:
Cake:

- ½ cup canola oil
- ½ teaspoon salt
- 1 cup buttermilk
- 1 cup hot coffee
- 1 cup white sugar
- 2 cups all-purpose flour
- 2 teaspoons baking powder
- 2 teaspoons instant coffee
- 3 eggs

Frosting:

- 1 cup heavy cream
- 2 cups dark chocolate chips
- 2 teaspoons instant coffee

Directions:

1. For the cake, combine the buttermilk, canola oil, hot coffee and eggs in a container.
2. Stir in the dry ingredients and mix thoroughly.
3. Pour the batter in a 9-inch round cake pan coated with baking paper.
4. Pre-heat the oven and bake at 350F for about fifty minutes.
5. When finished, transfer the chilled cake on a platter.
6. For the frosting, bring the cream to the boiling point in a saucepan. Put in the chocolate and stir until it melts completely. Stir in the coffee.
7. Cover the cake with chocolate coffee frosting and serve it fresh.

Nutritional Content of One Serving:
Calories: 371 | Fat: 19.6g | Protein: 5.8g | Carbohydrates: 47.6g

Chocolate Dulce De Leche Cake

Total Time Taken: 1 ¼ hours
Yield: 12 Servings
Ingredients:

- ½ cup butter, softened
- ½ cup canola oil
- ½ cup dulce de leche
- ½ cup sour cream
- ½ teaspoon salt
- 1 ¾ cups all-purpose flour
- 1 cup dark chocolate chips
- 1 cup white sugar
- 2 teaspoons baking powder
- 3 eggs

Directions:

1. Mix the butter and oil in a container. Put in the sugar and stir thoroughly until creamy.
2. Put in the eggs and sour cream and mix thoroughly.
3. Fold in the flour, baking powder and salt then put in the chocolate chips. Pour the batter in a 9-inch round cake pan coated with baking paper.
4. Drop spoonfuls of dulce de leche over the batter and preheat your oven and bake at 350F for about forty minutes or until a toothpick inserted into the center of the cake comes out clean.
5. *The cake tastes best chilled.*

Nutritional Content of One Serving:
Calories: 397 | Fat: 23.2g | Protein: 5.0g | Carbohydrates: 45.8g

Chocolate Fudge Cake

Total Time Taken: 1 ½ hours
Yield: 12 Servings
Ingredients:
Cake:

- ¼ cup cocoa powder
- ¼ teaspoon salt
- ½ cup dark chocolate chips
- 1 cup hot water
- ½ cup sour cream
- ½ teaspoon baking soda
- ¾ cup butter, softened

- 1 ½ teaspoons baking powder
- 1 ¾ cups all-purpose flour
- 1 cup dark brown sugar
- 2 eggs
- 2 tablespoons vegetable oil
- 1 teaspoon vanilla extract

Frosting:

- ½ cup cocoa powder
- 1 pinch salt
- 1 cup butter, softened
- 2 cups powdered sugar
- 2 tablespoons whole milk

Directions:

1. To prepare the cake, combine the chocolate chips, hot water and cocoa powder in a container.
2. In a separate container, combine the butter and sugar until creamy and pale. Stir in the eggs, one at a time, then put in the sour cream, vanilla and oil.
3. Mix the flour with baking powder, baking soda and salt then mix it with the butter mixture alternating it with the chocolate mixture. Begin and finish with flour.
4. Split the batter between two 9-inch circular cake pans covered with parchment paper.
5. Pre-heat the oven and bake at 350F for about half an hour.
6. Let cool and then take the cakes out of the pans and let them sit on the side you perform the next few steps.
7. For the frosting: combine the butter and powdered sugar for minimum five minutes until creamy and fluffy.
8. Put in the cocoa powder, salt and milk and stir thoroughly for another five minutes.
9. Use half of the frosting to fill the cake then garnish it with the half that is left over.
10. Serve immediately or place in your fridge until it is time to serve.

Nutritional Content of One Serving:

Calories: 517 | Fat: 34.2g | Protein: 4.8g | Carbohydrates: 52.9g

Chocolate Hazelnut Cake

Total Time Taken: 1 ¼ hours

Yield: 10 Servings

Ingredients:

Cake:

- ½ cup cocoa powder
- ½ teaspoon baking powder
- ½ teaspoon salt
- 1 cup all-purpose flour
- 1 cup ground hazelnuts
- 1 cup white sugar
- 6 eggs

Glaze:

- ½ cup heavy cream
- 1 cup dark chocolate chips

Directions:

1. To prepare the cake, combine the eggs with sugar until fluffy, minimum volume increases to twice what it was.
2. Fold in the flour, cocoa powder, baking powder, salt and hazelnuts then pour the batter in a 9-inch round cake pan coated with baking paper.
3. Preheat your oven and bake the cake for forty minutes or until a toothpick inserted in the center comes out clean.
4. Let the cake cool in the pan then move to a platter.
5. For the glaze, bring the cream to the boiling point then put in the chocolate and mix thoroughly.
6. Pour the warm glaze over the cake. Serve immediately or place in your refrigerator.

Nutritional Content of One Serving:

Calories: 292 | Fat: 13.3g | Protein: 7.4g | Carbohydrates: 41.6g

Chocolate Hazelnut Cake

Total Time Taken: 1 ¼ hours

Yield: 10 Servings

Ingredients:

- ¼ cup heavy cream
- ½ cup cherry jam
- ½ cup cocoa powder
- ½ cup white sugar
- ½ teaspoon baking soda
- ½ teaspoon salt
- 1 cup all-purpose flour
- 1 cup ground hazelnuts
- 1 teaspoon baking powder
- 2 whole eggs
- 6 egg yolks

Directions:

1. Mix the hazelnuts, flour, baking powder, baking soda and salt in a container. Put in the cocoa powder as well.
2. Mix the eggs, egg yolks and sugar in a container until thickened and fluffy. Stir in the cream and cherry jam.
3. Fold in the flour then spoon the cake in a 8-inch round cake pan coated with baking paper.
4. Pre-heat the oven and bake at 350F for around forty minutes or until a toothpick inserted into the center of the cake comes out clean.
5. The cake tastes best chilled.

Nutritional Content of One Serving:

Calories: 240 | Fat: 9.9g | Protein: 6.0g | Carbohydrates: 34.9g

Chocolate Mousse Cake

Total Time Taken: 1 ½ hours

Yield: 10 Servings

Ingredients:
Cake:
- ¼ cup cocoa powder
- ¼ cup heavy cream
- ¼ teaspoon salt
- ½ cup dark chocolate chips
- 1 cup all-purpose flour
- 1 cup buttermilk
- 1 egg
- 1 teaspoon baking powder

Chocolate mousse:
- ½ cup heavy cream, heated
- 1 cup dark chocolate chips
- 1 cup heavy cream, whipped

Directions:
1. For the cake, melt the cream and chocolate together in a heatproof container.
2. Stir in the remaining ingredients and stir for a few seconds to mix.
3. Pour the batter in a 9-inch round cake pan coated with baking paper.
4. Pre-heat the oven and bake at 350F for around forty minutes or until well risen and fragrant.
5. When finished, move the cake to a cake ring and place it on a platter.
6. For the chocolate mousse, combine the cream and chocolate chips in a container. Stir until melted and smooth. Let cool down.
7. Fold in the whipped cream then pour the mousse over the cake.
8. *Chill the cake before you serve.*

Nutritional Content of One Serving:
Calories: 223 | Fat: 13.6g | Protein: 4.7g | Carbohydrates: 24.7g

Chocolate Nutella Cake

Total Time Taken: 1 ½ hours
Yield: 10 Servings
Ingredients:
- ½ cup brewed coffee
- ½ cup canola oil
- ½ teaspoon salt
- 1 cup ground hazelnuts
- 1 cup Nutella
- 1 cup whole milk
- 1 teaspoon vanilla extract
- 2 cups all-purpose flour
- 2 eggs
- 2 tablespoons Kahlua
- 2 teaspoons baking powder

Directions:
1. Mix the ground hazelnuts, flour, baking powder and salt in a container.
2. Mix the eggs, milk, canola oil, Kahlua, vanilla and coffee in a separate container. Stir in the flour mixture then spoon the batter in a 9-inch round cake pan coated with baking paper.
3. Drop spoonfuls of Nutella over the batter and preheat your oven and bake at 350F for about forty minutes or until a toothpick inserted into the center of the cake comes out clean.
4. *The cake tastes best chilled.*

Nutritional Content of One Serving:
Calories: 295 | Fat: 18.5g | Protein: 5.8g | Carbohydrates: 25.4g

Chocolate Olive Oil Cake

Total Time Taken: 1 ¼ hours
Yield: 10 Servings
Ingredients:
- ¼ cup whole milk
- ¼ teaspoon salt
- ½ cup cocoa powder
- 1 cup all-purpose flour
- 1 cup white sugar
- 1 teaspoon baking powder
- 1 teaspoon orange zest
- 1 teaspoon vanilla extract
- 2 eggs
- 2/3 cup olive oil

Directions:
1. Mix the eggs with sugar until fluffy and pale. Stir in the vanilla and orange zest and mix thoroughly.
2. Put in the olive oil and milk then fold in the cocoa powder, flour, salt and baking powder.
3. Pour the batter in a 8-inch round cake pan coated with baking paper.
4. Pre-heat the oven and bake at 350F for forty minutes or until a toothpick inserted in the center comes out clean.
5. *The cake tastes best chilled.*

Nutritional Content of One Serving:
Calories: 263 | Fat: 15.2g | Protein: 3.4g | Carbohydrates: 32.6g

Chocolate Peanut Butter Bundt Cake

Total Time Taken: 1 ¼ hours
Yield: 10 Servings
Ingredients:
- ¼ cup whole milk
- ½ cup cocoa powder
- ½ teaspoon salt
- 1 ½ cups all-purpose flour
- 1 cup butter, softened
- 1 cup light brown sugar
- 1 cup sour cream
- 1 teaspoon baking powder
- 1 teaspoon baking soda
- 1 teaspoon vanilla extract
- 2/3 cup smooth peanut butter
- 3 eggs

Directions:
1. Mix the butter, sugar and vanilla in a container until fluffy and creamy.
2. Put in the eggs, one at a time, then mix in the sour cream and milk.
3. Fold in the flour, cocoa powder, baking powder, baking soda and salt.
4. Spoon half of the batter in a greased Bundt cake pan. Top with spoonfuls of peanut butter then cover with the rest of the batter.
5. Pre-heat the oven and bake at 350F for about forty minutes or until a toothpick inserted into the center of the cake comes out clean.
6. *The cake tastes best chilled.*

Nutritional Content of One Serving:
Calories: 470 | Fat: 34.1g | Protein: 9.8g | Carbohydrates: 35.9g

Chocolate Peppermint Cake

Total Time Taken: 1 ½ hours
Yield: 8 Servings
Ingredients:
Cake:
- ¼ teaspoon salt
- ½ cup butter, cubed
- ½ cup light brown sugar
- 1 cup all-purpose flour
- 1 cup dark chocolate chips
- 1 teaspoon baking powder
- 2 eggs
- 2 tablespoons cocoa powder

Glaze:
- ¼ cup heavy cream
- ¼ cup whole milk
- 1 pinch salt
- 3 tablespoons cocoa powder

Directions:
1. For the cake, combine the chocolate chips and butter in a heatproof container and place over a hot water bath. Melt them together until the desired smoothness is achieved.
2. Put in the sugar and eggs and mix thoroughly.
3. Stir in the flour, cocoa powder, baking powder and salt. Pour the batter in a 8-inch round cake pan coated with baking paper.
4. Pre-heat the oven and bake at 350F for about half an hour.
5. For the glaze, combine all the ingredients in a saucepan and place over low heat. Cook until it becomes thick.
6. Sprinkle the glaze over the cake and serve chilled.

Nutritional Content of One Serving:
Calories: 304 | Fat: 18.8g | Protein: 5.1g | Carbohydrates: 33.5g

Chocolate Pumpkin Cake

Total Time Taken: 1 hour
Yield: 10 Servings
Ingredients:
- ½ cup buttermilk
- ½ cup cocoa powder
- ½ cup sour cream
- ½ teaspoon ground star anise
- ½ teaspoon salt
- 1 cup butter, softened
- 1 cup light brown sugar
- 1 cup pumpkin puree
- 1 teaspoon baking powder
- 1 teaspoon baking soda
- 1 teaspoon ground cinnamon
- 1 teaspoon ground ginger
- 1 teaspoon vanilla extract
- 2 cups all-purpose flour
- 4 eggs

Directions:
1. Mix the butter and sugar in a container until fluffy and creamy.
2. Stir in the eggs, one at a time, then put in the vanilla, pumpkin puree, sour cream and buttermilk and mix thoroughly.
3. Fold in the dry ingredients then spoon the batter in a 10-inch round cake pan coated with baking paper.
4. Preheat your oven and bake the cake for about fifty minutes or until a toothpick inserted in the center comes out clean.
5. Let the cake cool in the pan and serve, sliced.

Nutritional Content of One Serving:
Calories: 385 | Fat: 23.6g | Protein: 6.9g | Carbohydrates: 39.6g

Cinnamon Chocolate Cake

Total Time Taken: 1 hour
Yield: 10 Servings
Ingredients:
- ½ cup buttermilk
- ½ cup cocoa powder
- ½ teaspoon salt
- 1 ½ cups white sugar
- 1 cup butter, softened
- 1 cup hot coffee
- 1 teaspoon cinnamon powder
- 1 teaspoon vanilla extract
- 2 cups all-purpose flour
- 2 teaspoons baking powder
- 3 eggs

Directions:
1. Mix the butter, sugar and cocoa powder in a container until creamy.

2. Stir in the eggs and vanilla and mix thoroughly.
3. Fold in the flour, baking powder and salt then put in the cinnamon, coffee and buttermilk and stir lightly.
4. Pour the batter in a 9-inch round cake pan coated with baking paper and bake for around forty minutes or until well risen and fragrant.
5. Let the cake cool in the pan before you serve.

Nutritional Content of One Serving:
Calories: 402 | Fat: 20.6g | Protein: 5.7g | Carbohydrates: 52.7g

Cinnamon Frosted Banana Cake

Total Time Taken: 1 ½ hours
Yield: 16 Servings
Ingredients:
Cake:

- ½ cup dark chocolate chips
- ½ teaspoon salt
- 1 cup canola oil
- 1 cup light brown sugar
- 1 cup sour cream
- 2 cups all-purpose flour
- 2 eggs
- 2 teaspoons baking powder
- 3 bananas, mashed

Cinnamon cream:

- ½ cup butter, softened
- 1 cup cream cheese
- 1 cup powdered sugar

Directions:

1. For the cake, combine the flour, baking powder and salt in a container.
2. In a separate container, combine the oil, sugar and eggs until fluffy and pale. Put in the bananas and sour cream and mix thoroughly then fold in the flour. Put in the chocolate chips too.
3. Spoon the batter in a 9-inch round cake pan and preheat your oven and bake at 350F for around forty minutes.
4. Let the cake cool in the pan then move to a platter.
5. For the frosting, combine the butter, cream cheese and sugar in a container for 5
6. minutes.
7. Cover the cake in frosting and serve it fresh.

Nutritional Content of One Serving:
Calories: 419 | Fat: 29.2g | Protein: 4.4g | Carbohydrates: 37.2g

Cinnamon Maple Pumpkin Cake

Total Time Taken: 1 ¼ hours
Yield: 10 Servings
Ingredients:

- ¼ teaspoon salt
- ½ cup canola oil
- ½ cup maple syrup
- ½ cup whole milk
- ½ teaspoon baking soda
- 1 ½ cups pumpkin puree
- 1 tablespoon cinnamon powder
- 1 teaspoon vanilla extract
- 2 ½ cups all-purpose flour
- 2 eggs
- 2 teaspoons baking powder
- 3/4 cup white sugar

Directions:

1. Mix the flour, baking powder, salt, baking soda and cinnamon in a container.
2. Mix the oil and sugar in a container for 2 minutes. Put in the eggs and mix thoroughly.
3. Stir in the pumpkin puree, vanilla and milk and mix thoroughly.
4. Fold in the flour mixture and mix using a spatula. Pour the batter in a 9-inch round cake pan coated with baking paper.
5. Pre-heat the oven and bake at 350F for about forty-five minutes or until a toothpick inserted into the center of the cake comes out clean.
6. *The cake tastes best chilled.*

Nutritional Content of One Serving:
Calories: 342 | Fat: 12.6g | Protein: 5.1g | Carbohydrates: 53.5g

Cinnamon Streusel Raspberry Cake

Total Time Taken: 1 ¼ hours
Yield: 12 Servings
Ingredients:
Cake:

- ¼ cup canola oil
- ½ cup butter, softened
- ½ teaspoon salt
- ¾ cup whole milk
- 1 cup fresh raspberries Cinnamon
- 1 teaspoon vanilla extract
- 2 cups all-purpose flour
- 2 eggs
- 2 teaspoons baking powder

Streusel:

- ¼ cup light brown sugar
- ½ cup all-purpose flour
- ½ cup butter, chilled
- 1 pinch salt
- 1 teaspoon cinnamon powder

Directions:

1. To prepare the cake, sift the flour, baking powder and salt in a container.
2. In a separate container, combine the butter, oil and eggs until creamy. Stir in the milk and vanilla then fold in the flour.

3. Put in the raspberries then spoon the batter in a 8x8-inch cake pan coated with baking paper.
4. Make the cinnamon by mixing all the ingredients in a container until grainy.
5. Spread the streusel over the cake and preheat your oven and bake at 350F for about forty minutes or until fragrant and golden brown.
6. Let the cake cool in the pan and serve, sliced.

Nutritional Content of One Serving:
Calories: 309 | Fat: 21.4g | Protein: 4.4g | Carbohydrates: 25.3g

Citrus Poppy Seed Bundt Cake

Total Time Taken: 1 ¼ hours
Yield: 12 Servings
Ingredients:

- ½ cup butter, softened
- ½ cup canola oil
- ½ teaspoon salt
- 1 cup sour cream
- 1 cup white sugar
- 1 lemon, zested and juiced
- 1 lime, zested and juiced
- 2 cups all-purpose flour
- 2 eggs
- 2 tablespoons poppy seeds
- 2 teaspoons baking powder

Directions:

1. Mix the canola oil, butter and sugar in a container until creamy and pale.
2. Stir in the eggs and mix thoroughly then put in the sour cream.
3. Combine in the lime zest and juice, as well as the lemon zest and juice.
4. Fold in the remaining ingredients then spoon the batter in a greased Bundt cake pan.
5. Pre-heat the oven and bake at 350F for about forty minutes or until it rises significantly and starts to appear golden-brown.
6. Let the cake cool in the pan before you serve.

Nutritional Content of One Serving:
Calories: 350 | Fat: 22.4g | Protein: 4.1g | Carbohydrates: 35.2g

Classic Fruit Cake

Total Time Taken: 2 hours
Yield: 16 Servings
Ingredients:

- ½ cup dates, pitted and chopped
- ½ cup dried apricots, chopped
- ½ cup dried cranberries
- ½ cup dried pineapple, chopped
- ½ cup fresh orange juice
- ½ cup sliced almonds
- ½ teaspoon baking powder
- ½ teaspoon salt
- 1 cup brandy
- 1 cup butter, softened
- 1 cup golden raisins
- 1 cup light brown sugar
- 1 cup sultanas
- 1 teaspoon baking soda
- 2 cups all-purpose flour
- 2 tablespoons orange zest
- 4 eggs

Directions:

1. Mix the dried fruits and brandy in a container. Allow to soak up for minimum an hour.
2. Mix the butter and sugar in a container until creamy and pale.
3. Put in the orange zest and orange juice and mix thoroughly then mix in the eggs, one at a time.
4. Fold in the flour, almonds, baking soda, baking powder and salt.
5. Put in the fruits and stir lightly using a spatula.
6. Spoon the batter in a 9-inch round cake pan coated with baking paper.
7. Pre-heat the oven and bake at 350F for 55-60 minutes. The cake is done when a toothpick inserted in the center comes out clean.
8. Let the cake cool in the pan then serve, sliced.

Nutritional Content of One Serving:
Calories: 290 | Fat: 14.4g | Protein: 4.4g | Carbohydrates: 37.2g

Coconut Carrot Bundt Cake

Total Time Taken: 1 ¼ hours
Yield: 10 Servings
Ingredients:

- ½ cup coconut milk
- ½ cup crushed pineapple
- ½ teaspoon salt
- 1 ¼ cups all-purpose flour
- 1 cup canola oil
- 1 cup coconut flakes
- 1 cup light brown sugar
- 1 cup shredded coconut
- 1 tablespoon orange zest
- 1 teaspoon vanilla extract
- 2 cups grated carrots
- 2 teaspoons baking powder
- 4 eggs

Directions:

1. Mix the eggs and sugar in a container until volume increases to twice what it was.
2. Stir in the oil and vanilla then put in the orange zest, coconut, carrots, pineapple and coconut milk.

3. Fold in the flour, baking powder and salt then pour the batter in a 9-inch round cake pan coated with baking paper.
4. Pre-heat the oven and bake at 350F for about forty minutes or until a toothpick inserted in the center comes out clean.
5. Let the cake cool in the pan and serve, sliced.

Nutritional Content of One Serving:
Calories: 430 | Fat: 31.9g | Protein: 4.9g | Carbohydrates: 33.3g

Coconut Raspberry Cake

Total Time Taken: 1 hour
Yield: 8 Servings
Ingredients:

- ¼ cup coconut milk
- ½ cup butter, softened
- ½ cup coconut oil, melted
- ½ teaspoon salt
- 1 3/4 cups all-purpose flour
- 1 cup fresh raspberries
- 1 cup shredded coconut
- 1 cup white sugar
- 1 teaspoon baking soda
- 4 eggs

Directions:
1. **Mix** the flour, shredded coconut, salt and baking soda in a container.
2. In a separate container, mix the butter, coconut oil and sugar in a container. **Stir thoroughly to mix** until fluffy then put in the eggs, one at a time, and **mix thoroughly**.
3. **Stir in** the coconut oil then fold in the dry ingredients.
4. Spoon the batter in a 9-inch cake pan coated with baking paper.
5. Top with fresh raspberries and preheat your oven and bake at 350F for around forty minutes or **until a golden-brown colour is achieved and it rises significantly.**
6. **The cake tastes best chilled**.

Nutritional Content of One Serving:
Calories: 505 | Fat: 32.8g | Protein: 6.4g | Carbohydrates: 49.8g

Cranberry Upside Down Cake

Total Time Taken: 1 hour
Yield: 10 Servings
Ingredients:

- ¼ teaspoon salt
- ½ cup butter, melted and chilled
- 1 ½ cups all-purpose flour
- ½ cup light brown sugar
- ½ teaspoon baking powder
- 1 cup fresh cranberries
- 1 cup white sugar
- 1 teaspoon vanilla extract
- 6 eggs

Directions:
1. Position the cranberries at the bottom of a round cake pan. Drizzle with brown sugar.
2. Mix the eggs and sugar in a container until fluffy and volume increases to twice what it was.
3. Stir in the butter and stir lightly.
4. Fold in the flour, baking powder and salt.
5. Pour the batter over the cranberries and preheat your oven and bake at 350F for about forty minutes or until it rises significantly and starts to appear golden-brown.
6. When finished, flip the cake upside down on a platter and serve chilled.

Nutritional Content of One Serving:
Calories: 297 | Fat: 12.0g | Protein: 5.4g | Carbohydrates: 42.8g

Cream Bundt Cake

Total Time Taken: 1 hour
Yield: 10 Servings
Ingredients:

- ½ teaspoon salt
- 1 ½ cups heavy cream
- 1 cup white sugar
- 1 teaspoon vanilla extract
- 2 cups all-purpose flour
- 2 teaspoons baking powder
- 3 eggs

Directions:
1. Sift the flour, baking powder and salt.
2. Whip the heavy cream on moderate speed until soft peaks form. Carry on whipping until firm.
3. Stir in the eggs, one at a time, then put in the sugar and mix thoroughly.
4. Fold in the flour then spoon the batter in a Bundt cake pan lined using butter.
5. Pre-heat the oven and bake at 350F for around forty minutes or until a toothpick inserted in the center comes out clean.
6. Let the cake cool in the pan for about ten minutes then move to a platter.

Nutritional Content of One Serving:
Calories: 249 | Fat: 8.2g | Protein: 4.6g | Carbohydrates: 40.2g

Cream Cheese Apple Cake

Total Time Taken: 1 ¼ hours
Yield: 10 Servings
Ingredients:

- ½ cup canola oil
- ½ teaspoon salt
- 1 ½ cups white sugar
- 1 cup cream cheese

- 1 teaspoon vanilla extract
- 2 cups all-purpose flour
- 2 red apples, peeled, cored and diced
- 2 teaspoons baking powder
- 3 eggs

Directions:

1. Mix the cream cheese, canola oil and sugar in a container until pale and creamy.
2. Put in the eggs and mix thoroughly then mix in the vanilla, followed by the rest of the dry ingredients.
3. Combine in the apples then spoon the batter in a 9-inch round cake pan coated with baking paper.
4. Pre-heat the oven and bake at 350F for about fifty minutes or until it rises significantly and starts to appear golden-brown.
5. Let the cake cool in the pan before you serve.

Nutritional Content of One Serving:

Calories: 421 | Fat: 20.6g | Protein: 6.1g | Carbohydrates: 55.4g

Cream Cheese Pumpkin Cake

Total Time Taken: 1 ¼ hours

Yield: 14 Servings

Ingredients:

Cake:

- ½ teaspoon ground cloves
- ½ teaspoon ground ginger
- ½ teaspoon salt
- 1 ½ cups pumpkin puree
- 1 cup canola oil
- 1 teaspoon cinnamon powder
- 1 teaspoon ground ginger
- 2 cups all-purpose flour
- 2 cups white sugar
- 2 teaspoons baking soda
- 4 eggs

Cream cheese frosting:

- ½ cup butter, softened
- 1 cup cream cheese
- 1 cup powdered sugar

Directions:

1. For the cake, combine the pumpkin puree, sugar, eggs and canola oil in a container.
2. Stir in the remaining ingredients and stir until incorporated, don't over mix it!
3. Pour the batter in a 10-inch round cake pan coated with baking paper.
4. Pre-heat the oven and bake at 350F for about forty-five minutes or until it rises significantly and starts to appear golden-brown.
5. Let the cake cool in the pan then move to a platter.
6. For the frosting, combine all the ingredients in a container. Spread the frosting over the cake and serve fresh or place in your refrigerator.

Nutritional Content of One Serving:

Calories: 487 | Fat: 29.5g | Protein: 5.0g | Carbohydrates: 53.6g

Cream Cheese Pumpkin Cake

Total Time Taken: 1 ¼ hours

Yield: 14 Servings

Ingredients:

Cake:

- ½ teaspoon ground cloves
- ½ teaspoon ground ginger
- ½ teaspoon salt
- 1 ½ cups pumpkin puree
- 1 cup canola oil
- 1 teaspoon cinnamon powder
- 1 teaspoon ground ginger
- 2 cups all-purpose flour
- 2 cups white sugar
- 2 teaspoons baking soda
- 4 eggs

Cream cheese frosting:

- ½ cup butter, softened
- 1 cup cream cheese
- 1 cup powdered sugar

Directions:

1. For the cake, combine the pumpkin puree, sugar, eggs and canola oil in a container.
2. Stir in the remaining ingredients and stir until incorporated, don't over mix it!
3. Pour the batter in a 10-inch round cake pan coated with baking paper.
4. Pre-heat the oven and bake at 350F for about forty-five minutes or until it rises significantly and starts to appear golden-brown.
5. Let the cake cool in the pan then move to a platter.
6. For the frosting, combine all the ingredients in a container. Spread the frosting over the cake and serve fresh or place in your refrigerator.

Nutritional Content of One Serving:

Calories: 487 | Fat: 29.5g | Protein: 5.0g | Carbohydrates: 53.6g

Dark Chocolate Coffee Cake

Total Time Taken: 1 ¼ hours

Yield: 8 Servings

Ingredients:

- ¼ cup cocoa powder
- ¼ cup sour cream
- ½ cup light brown sugar
- ½ teaspoon salt
- 1 ½ cups all-purpose flour
- 1 teaspoon baking powder

- 1 teaspoon vanilla extract
- 3 oz. dark chocolate, melted
- 4 eggs
- 4 tablespoons butter, softened

Directions:

1. Mix the butter and chocolate, then mix in the eggs, sugar, vanilla and sour cream.
2. Fold in the flour, cocoa powder, baking powder and salt and stir lightly using a spatula.
3. Spoon the batter in a 9-inch round cake pan and preheat your oven and bake at 350F for around forty minutes or until it passes the toothpicks test.
4. Let the cake cool in the pan before you serve.

Nutritional Content of One Serving:

Calories: 282 | Fat: 13.2g | Protein: 6.8g | Carbohydrates: 35.4g

Dark Rum Pecan Cake

Total Time Taken: 1 ¼ hours
Yield: 10 Servings
Ingredients:
Cake:

- ¼ cup sour cream
- ½ cup light brown sugar
- ½ cup white sugar
- ½ teaspoon baking powder
- ½ teaspoon salt
- ¾ cup butter, softened
- 1 ½ cups all-purpose flour
- 1 cup ground pecans
- 1 teaspoon baking soda
- 3 eggs

Glaze:

- 1 cup powdered sugar
- 2 tablespoons dark rum

Directions:

1. To prepare the cake, combine the flour, pecans, baking soda, baking powder and salt in a container.
2. In a separate container, combine the butter and sugars until creamy. Put in the eggs, one after another, then mix in the sour cream and mix thoroughly.
3. Fold in the flour mixture then spoon the batter in a 9-inch round cake pan covered with parchment paper.
4. Pre-heat the oven and bake at 350F for around forty minutes until a golden-brown colour is achieved and well risen then transfer the cake on a platter and allow to cool.
5. For the glaze, combine the sugar with dark rum. Sprinkle the glaze over the chilled cake and serve immediately.

Nutritional Content of One Serving:

Calories: 350 | Fat: 17.5g | Protein: 4.1g | Carbohydrates: 44.0g

Decadent Chocolate Cake

Total Time Taken: 1 hour
Yield: 10 Servings
Ingredients:

- ¼ cup all-purpose flour
- ½ cup cocoa powder
- ½ teaspoon salt
- 1 cup butter, softened
- 2/3 cup white sugar
- 3 cups dark chocolate chips
- 6 eggs, separated

Directions:

1. Melt the butter and chocolate chips in a heatproof container over a hot water bath.
2. Mix the egg yolks and sugar in a container until fluffy and pale.
3. Stir in the melted chocolate, then put in the cocoa powder, flour and salt.
4. Whip the egg whites until fluffy and firm. Fold the meringue into the batter then pour the batter in a 9-inch round cake pan.
5. Pre-heat the oven and bake at 350F for around forty minutes or until well risen.
6. *The cake tastes best chilled.*

Nutritional Content of One Serving:

Calories: 439 | Fat: 31.2g | Protein: 7.0g | Carbohydrates: 42.3g

Devils Bundt Cake

Total Time Taken: 1 ¼ hours
Yield: 14 Servings
Ingredients:
Cake:

- ¼ teaspoon baking soda
- ½ teaspoon salt
- 1 ½ cups white sugar
- 1 cup butter, softened
- 1 cup cocoa powder
- 1 cup hot water
- 1 cup sour cream
- 1 cup white chocolate chips
- 2 ½ cups all-purpose flour
- 2 teaspoons baking powder
- 4 eggs

Glaze:

- ½ cup heavy cream
- ¾ cup dark chocolate chips

Directions:

1. For the cake, combine the cocoa powder, water and sour cream in a container.
2. In a separate container, sift the flour, baking powder, baking soda and salt.

3. Mix the butter and sugar in a container until fluffy. Put in the eggs, one at a time and mix thoroughly.
4. Stir in the cocoa powder mixture then fold in the flour.
5. Put in the chocolate chips then spoon the batter in a Bundt cake lined using butter.
6. Preheat your oven and bake the cake for about forty minutes or until a toothpick inserted in the center comes out clean.
7. Let the cake cool in the pan then move to a platter.
8. For the glaze, combine the two ingredients in a heatproof container and place over low heat. Melt them together then sprinkle the glaze over the cake.
9. Serve immediately or place in your refrigerator.

Nutritional Content of One Serving:
Calories: 456 | Fat: 26.1g | Protein: 6.9g | Carbohydrates: 54.6g

Duo Bundt Cake

Total Time Taken: 1 ¼ hours
Yield: 14 Servings
Ingredients:

- ¼ cup cocoa powder
- ¼ cup hot water
- ½ cup butter, softened
- ½ cup cream cheese
- ½ teaspoon baking soda
- ½ teaspoon salt
- 1 cup buttermilk
- 2 cups white sugar
- 2 teaspoons baking powder
- 3 cups all-purpose flour
- 3 eggs
- 4 oz. dark chocolate, melted

Directions:
1. Mix the butter and sugar in a container until creamy and fluffy.
2. Stir in the chocolate and eggs and mix thoroughly, then put in the cream cheese.
3. Sift the flour, baking powder, baking soda and salt then fold it in the batter.
4. Divide the batter in half. Combine one half with the cocoa powder and hot water.
5. Spoon the white batter in a greased Bundt cake pan.
6. Top with the cocoa batter and preheat your oven and bake at 350F for about fifty minutes or until well risen and it passes the toothpick test.
7. Let the cake cool in the pan then move to a platter.

Nutritional Content of One Serving:
Calories: 360 | Fat: 13.4g | Protein: 6.1g | Carbohydrates: 56.1g

Fluffy Pear Bundt Cake

Total Time Taken: 1 ¼ hours
Yield: 14 Servings
Ingredients:

- ½ cup whole milk
- ½ teaspoon salt
- 1 ½ cups white sugar
- 1 cup canola oil
- 1 teaspoon vanilla extract
- 2 teaspoons baking powder
- 2 teaspoons pumpkin pie spice
- 3 cups all-purpose flour
- 3 eggs
- 3 pears, peeled, cored and diced

Directions:
1. Mix the flour, baking powder, salt and pumpkin pie spice in a container.
2. In a separate container, combine the canola oil with sugar and eggs until volume increases to twice what it was.
3. Put in the vanilla extract and milk then fold in the flour, followed by the pears.
4. Spoon the batter in a greased Bundt cake pan and preheat your oven and bake at 350F for about fifty minutes or until a toothpick comes out clean after being inserted into the center of the cake.
5. Let the cake cool in the pan then serve, sliced.

Nutritional Content of One Serving:
Calories: 363 | Fat: 17.1g | Protein: 4.4g | Carbohydrates: 49.7g

French Apple Cake

Total Time Taken: 1 ¼ hours
Yield: 8 Servings
Ingredients:

- ¼ cup brandy
- ¼ teaspoon salt
- ½ cup butter, softened
- ½ teaspoon cinnamon powder
- 1 ½ cups all-purpose flour
- 1 cup light brown sugar
- 1 teaspoon baking powder
- 2 eggs
- 3 red apples, peeled, cored and sliced

Directions:
1. Sift the flour, baking powder and salt in a container.
2. Mix the eggs, sugar, brandy and butter in a container until fluffy and pale.
3. Fold in the flour then spoon the batter in a 8-inch round cake pan.

4. Top with apple slices and preheat your oven and bake at 350F for around forty minutes or until a golden-brown colour is achieved and it rises significantly.

5. *The cake tastes best chilled.*

Nutritional Content of One Serving:
Calories: 315 | Fat: 12.9g | Protein: 4.1g | Carbohydrates: 45.5g

Fruit and Brandy Cake

Total Time Taken: 1 ½ hours
Yield: 16 Servings
Ingredients:

- ¼ cup black treacle
- ¼ cup candied ginger, chopped
- ¼ cup honey
- ½ cup dried apricots, chopped
- ½ cup dried pineapple, chopped
- ½ cup golden syrup
- 1 cup brandy
- 1 cup butter, softened
- 1 cup dark brown sugar
- 1 cup golden raisins
- 1 cup heavy cream
- 1 teaspoon baking soda
- 1 teaspoon lemon zest
- 1 teaspoon orange zest
- 11 cup dried black currants
- 3 cups all-purpose flour
- 6 eggs

Directions:

1. Mix the dried fruits with brandy in a container and allow to soak up for a few hours, preferably overnight.
2. Mix the golden syrup, treacle, honey, brown sugar, cream, butter, lemon zest and orange zest in a container until creamy.
3. Stir in the eggs, one at a time, then put in the flour. and baking soda.
4. Fold in the dried fruits and stir lightly using a spatula.
5. Spoon the batter in a 10-inch round cake pan , preheat your oven and bake at 330F for an hour or until a toothpick comes out clean after being inserted into the center of the cake. If the toothpick is not clean, continue baking for 10 additional minutes and check again.
6. Let the cake cool in the pan then move to a platter and slice.

Nutritional Content of One Serving:
Calories: 450 | Fat: 16.3g | Protein: 5.2g | Carbohydrates: 73.3g

Fruity Bundt Cake

Total Time Taken: 1 ¼ hours
Yield: 12 Servings
Ingredients:

- ¼ cup dried apricots, chopped
- ¼ cup golden raisins
- ½ cup candied cherries, chopped
- ½ cup chopped almonds
- ½ cup chopped pecans
- 1 ½ cups white sugar
- 1 ½ teaspoons baking powder
- 1 cup butter, softened
- 1 cup cream cheese, room temperature
- 1 teaspoon vanilla extract
- 2 cups all-purpose flour
- 4 eggs

Directions:

1. Mix the cream cheese, butter and sugar in a container until fluffy and creamy.
2. Stir in the eggs, one at a time, then put in the eggs and vanilla.
3. Stir thoroughly to mix then fold in the rest of the ingredients.
4. Spoon the batter in a greased Bundt cake pan and preheat your oven and bake at 350F for about forty minutes or until it rises significantly and starts to appear golden-brown.
5. Let the cake cool in the pan before you serve.

Nutritional Content of One Serving:
Calories: 447 | Fat: 26.6g | Protein: 6.8g | Carbohydrates: 48.0g

Fudgy Chocolate Cake

Total Time Taken: 1 hour
Yield: 10 Servings
Ingredients:

- ½ cup butter, melted
- ½ cup cocoa powder
- ½ cup sour cream
- ½ teaspoon baking soda
- ½ teaspoon salt
- 1 3/4 cups all-purpose flour
- 1 cup hot coffee
- 1 cup white sugar
- 1 teaspoon baking powder
- 2 eggs
- 4 oz. dark chocolate, melted

Directions:

1. Mix the butter and chocolate in a container. Stir in the coffee, eggs and sour cream, as well as sugar.
2. Stir thoroughly to mix then fold in the remaining ingredients.
3. Spoon the batter in a 9-inch round cake pan , preheat your oven and bake at 330F for about fifty minutes.
4. Let the cake cool in the pan before you serve.

Nutritional Content of One Serving:
Calories: 344 | Fat: 16.6g | Protein: 5.5g | Carbohydrates: 46.6g

Fudgy Chocolate Cake

Total Time Taken: 1 hour
Yield: 10 Servings
Ingredients:

- ¼ teaspoon salt
- ½ cup cocoa powder
- ¾ cup all-purpose flour
- 1 cup butter
- 1 cup ground walnuts
- 1 cup white sugar
- 2 cups dark chocolate chips
- 3 eggs

Directions:

1. Mix the chocolate chips and butter in a container and place over a hot water bath. Melt it over heat until the desired smoothness is achieved.
2. Put in the sugar and mix thoroughly then mix in the eggs.
3. Fold in the flour, cocoa powder, salt and walnuts then spoon the batter in a 8- inch round cake pan coated with baking paper.
4. Pre-heat the oven and bake at 350F for a little more than half an hour.
5. Let the cake cool in the pan before you serve.

Nutritional Content of One Serving:
Calories: 490 | Fat: 34.1g | Protein: 8.2g | Carbohydrates: 46.9g

Funfetti Cake

Total Time Taken: 1 hour
Yield: 8 Servings
Ingredients:

- ¼ cup butter, melted
- ½ cup canola oil
- ½ cup funfetti sprinkles
- ½ cup whole milk
- ½ teaspoon salt
- 1 ½ cups all-purpose flour
- 1 ½ teaspoons baking powder
- 1 cup white sugar
- 1 teaspoon vanilla extract
- 3 eggs

Directions:

1. Mix the flour, baking powder, salt and sprinkles in a container.
2. In a separate container, mix the canola oil, butter and sugar and mix thoroughly. Put in the eggs and stir thoroughly for five minutes.
3. Stir in the vanilla and milk and mix thoroughly then pour this mixture over the dry ingredients and stir lightly.
4. Spoon the batter in a 9-inch cake pan coated with baking paper and preheat your oven and bake at 350F for around forty minutes.
5. Let the cake cool in the pan and serve, sliced.

Nutritional Content of One Serving:
Calories: 392 | Fat: 21.8g | Protein: 5.1g | Carbohydrates: 46.0g

Ganache Chocolate Cake

Total Time Taken: 1 ¼ hours
Yield: 8 Servings
Ingredients:
Cake:

- ¼ cup butter, melted and cooled **Ganache:**
- ¼ cup cocoa powder
- ¼ teaspoon salt
- ¾ cup all-purpose flour
- 1 cup dark chocolate, chopped
- 1 teaspoon baking powder
- 1 teaspoon vanilla extract
- 2/3 cup heavy cream
- 6 eggs, room temperature
- 2/3 cup white sugar

Directions:

1. To prepare the cake, combine the eggs, sugar and vanilla in the container of your stand mixer for about five to seven minutes until its volume increases to almost three times it was.
2. Fold in the flour, cocoa powder, salt and baking powder with the help of a wooden spoon or spatula, being cautious not to deflate the eggs.
3. Progressively fold in the melted butter.
4. Pour the batter in a 10-inch cake pan coated with baking paper and preheat your oven and bake at 350F for around forty minutes.
5. Let cool in the pan then move to a platter.
6. For the ganache, bring the cream to the boiling point then turn off heat and mix in the chocolate. Stir until melted and smooth then let cool to room temperature.
7. Spoon the ganache over the cake and serve immediately.

Nutritional Content of One Serving:
Calories: 358 | Fat: 19.4g | Protein: 7.7g | Carbohydrates: 40.5g

German Fruit Bundt Cake

Total Time Taken: 1 ¼ hours
Yield: 10 Servings
Ingredients:

- ¼ cup dark brown sugar
- ¼ cup dried cranberries
- ¼ cup golden raisins
- ½ teaspoon salt
- 1 cup butter, softened

- 1 cup white sugar
- 1 teaspoon cinnamon powder
- 2 cups all-purpose flour
- 2 eggs
- 2 pears, peeled, cored and diced
- 2 teaspoons baking powder

Directions:

1. Mix the flour, baking powder, salt and cinnamon in a container.
2. In a separate container, mix the butter with the sugars and mix thoroughly. Stir in the eggs, one at a time and mix thoroughly.
3. Fold in the flour mixture then put in the pears, raisins and cranberries.
4. Spoon the batter in a Bundt cake pan lined using butter and preheat your oven and bake the cake at 350F for around forty minutes or until a golden-brown colour is achieved and it passes the toothpick test.
5. Let the cake cool down and serve, sliced.

Nutritional Content of One Serving:
Calories: 393 | Fat: 19.6g | Protein: 4.1g | Carbohydrates: 52.7g

Ginger Sweet Potato Cake

Total Time Taken: 1 ½ hours
Yield: 10 Servings
Ingredients:

- ½ teaspoon baking soda
- ½ teaspoon salt
- ¾ cup canola oil
- 1 3/4 cups all-purpose flour
- 1 cup light brown sugar
- 1 cup sweet potato puree
- 1 tablespoon orange zest
- 1 teaspoon baking powder
- 1 teaspoon cinnamon powder
- 1 teaspoon vanilla extract
- 4 eggs

Directions:

1. Mix the sweet potato puree with the orange zest, canola oil, eggs, brown sugar and vanilla in a container.
2. Fold in the remaining ingredients then spoon the batter in a 9-inch round cake pan coated with baking paper.
3. Preheat your oven and bake the cake for around forty minutes or until a toothpick comes out clean after being inserted into the center of the cake.
4. Let the cake cool in the pan and serve, sliced.

Nutritional Content of One Serving:
Calories: 332 | Fat: 18.4g | Protein: 5.0g | Carbohydrates: 37.4g

Ginger Whole Orange Cake

Total Time Taken: 1 ¼ hours
Yield: 10 Servings
Ingredients:
Cake:

- ½ teaspoon salt
- 1 cup butter, softened
- 1 cup powdered sugar
- 1 cup white sugar
- 1 tablespoon orange juice
- 1 teaspoon grated ginger **Icing:**
- 1 teaspoon orange zest
- 1 whole orange
- 2 cups all-purpose flour
- 2 tablespoons dark brown sugar
- 2 teaspoons baking powder
- 4 eggs

Directions:

1. To prepare the cake, place the orange in a saucepan and cover it with water. Cook for about half an hour then drain well and place in a food processor. Pulse until the desired smoothness is achieved. Put in the ginger and mix thoroughly. Place aside.
2. Mix the butter with the sugars in a container until creamy and fluffy. Stir in the eggs, one at a time and mix thoroughly.
3. Fold in the flour, baking powder and salt, alternating it with the orange mixture.
4. Spoon the batter in a 9-inch round cake pan coated with baking paper and preheat your oven and bake at 350F for about forty minutes or until a toothpick comes out clean after being inserted into the center of the cake.
5. Let the cake cool then move it to a platter.
6. For the icing, combine all the ingredients in a container and sprinkle it over the chilled cake. Serve immediately.

Nutritional Content of One Serving:
Calories: 430 | Fat: 21.1g | Protein: 5.8g | Carbohydrates: 56.2g

Gingerbread Chocolate Cake

Total Time Taken: 1 ¼ hours
Yield: 10 Servings
Ingredients:

- ½ cup butter, softened
- ½ cup cocoa powder
- ½ cup sour cream
- ½ teaspoon ground cloves
- ½ teaspoon ground ginger
- ½ teaspoon ground star anise
- ½ teaspoon salt
- 1 ½ cups white sugar
- 1 teaspoon cinnamon powder
- 1 teaspoon orange zest
- 2 cups all-purpose flour
- 2 teaspoons baking powder

- 3 eggs
- 4 oz. dark chocolate, melted

Directions:

1. Mix the butter with sugar until creamy. Put in the eggs, one at a time, then mix in the melted chocolate and sour cream.
2. Fold in the flour, cocoa powder, baking powder, salt and spices.
3. Spoon the batter in a 9-icnh round cake pan coated with baking paper.
4. Pre-heat the oven and bake at 350F for forty minutes or until it rises completely and is aromatic.
5. Let the cake cool in the pan and serve, sliced.

Nutritional Content of One Serving:

Calories: 402 | Fat: 17.1g | Protein: 6.4g | Carbohydrates: 59.6g

Gingersnap Pumpkin Bundt Cake

Total Time Taken: 1 ¼ hours

Yield: 12 Servings

Ingredients:

- ¼ cup canola oil
- ½ cup butter, softened
- ½ teaspoon salt
- 1 ½ cups pumpkin puree
- 1 cup white sugar
- 1 teaspoon vanilla extract
- 2 cups all-purpose flour
- 2 tablespoons dark brown sugar
- 2 teaspoons baking powder
- 3 eggs
- 6 gingersnaps, crushed

Directions:

1. Mix the butter, oil and sugars in a container until light and creamy.
2. Stir in the eggs, one at a time, then put in the pumpkin and vanilla and mix thoroughly.
3. Fold in the flour, baking powder and salt then put in the crushed gingersnaps.
4. Spoon the batter in a greased Bundt cake pan and preheat your oven and bake at 350F for 45 minutes or until a toothpick comes out clean after being inserted into the center of the cake.
5. Let cool in the pan then move to a platter.

Nutritional Content of One Serving:

Calories: 350 | Fat: 16.1g | Protein: 5.0g | Carbohydrates: 48.0g

Graham Cracker Cake

Total Time Taken: 1 ¼ hours

Yield: 10 Servings

Ingredients:

- ¼ cup dark brown sugar
- ½ cup heavy cream
- ½ teaspoon baking powder
- ½ teaspoon cinnamon powder
- ½ teaspoon salt
- ¾ cup butter, softened
- 1 cup graham cracker crumbs
- 1 cup white sugar
- 2 cups all-purpose flour
- 2 teaspoons baking powder
- 3 eggs

Directions:

1. Mix the graham cracker crumbs, flour, baking powder, baking soda, salt and cinnamon in a container.
2. In another container, combine the butter and sugars until creamy and light.
3. Stir in the eggs, one after another, and mix thoroughly then put in the cream.
4. Fold in the flour mixture then pour the batter in a 10-inch round cake pan coated with baking paper.
5. Bake for about forty-five minutes in the preheated oven at 350F or until a toothpick comes out clean after being inserted into the center of the cake.
6. Let the cake cool in the pan and serve, sliced.

Nutritional Content of One Serving:

Calories: 380 | Fat: 18.4g | Protein: 5.0g | Carbohydrates: 50.4g

Graham Cracker Pumpkin Cake

Total Time Taken: 1 ¼ hours

Yield: 12 Servings

Ingredients:

- ¼ cup dark brown sugar
- ½ cup butter, softened
- ½ cup whole milk
- ½ teaspoon salt
- 1 ¼ cups pumpkin puree
- 1 ½ cups graham crackers
- 1 cup all-purpose flour
- 1 cup light brown sugar
- 2 teaspoons baking powder
- 4 eggs

Directions:

1. Mix the butter with the sugars in a container until creamy and fluffy.
2. Stir in the eggs, one at a time, then put in the pumpkin puree and milk.
3. Put in the rest of the ingredients and mix thoroughly using a spatula.
4. Pour the batter in a greased Bundt cake pan and preheat your oven and bake at 350F for forty minutes or until it rises significantly and starts to appear golden-brown.

5. Let the cake cool in the pan before you serve.

Nutritional Content of One Serving:
Calories: 244 | Fat: 10.7g | Protein: 4.4g | Carbohydrates: 33.9g

Grand Marnier Infused Loaf Cake

Total Time Taken: 2 hours
Yield: 14 Servings
Ingredients:

- ¼ cup grand Marnier
- ½ cup butter, softened
- ½ cup whole milk
- ½ teaspoon baking soda
- ½ teaspoon salt
- 1 ½ cups white sugar
- 1 cup cream cheese
- 1 cup dried cranberries
- 1 teaspoon vanilla extract
- 2 teaspoons baking powder
- 3 cups all-purpose flour
- 4 eggs

Directions:
1. Mix the cranberries and Grand Marnier in a jar and allow to soak up for an hour.
2. Mix the flour with baking powder, baking soda and salt.
3. Mix the butter, cream cheese and sugar in a container until fluffy.
4. Stir in the eggs, one at a time, then put in the vanilla and milk.
5. Fold in the flour mixture and stir until incorporated.
6. Put in the cranberries.
7. Spoon the batter in a large loaf pan coated with baking paper.
8. Pre-heat the oven and bake at 350F for about fifty minutes or until a toothpick inserted in the center comes out clean.
9. Let the cake cool in the pan then serve, sliced.

Nutritional Content of One Serving:
Calories: 336 | Fat: 14.1g | Protein: 6.0g | Carbohydrates: 43.9g

Grand Marnier Infused Loaf Cake

Total Time Taken: 2 hours
Yield: 14 Servings
Ingredients:

- ¼ cup grand Marnier
- ½ cup butter, softened
- ½ cup whole milk
- ½ teaspoon baking soda
- ½ teaspoon salt
- 1 ½ cups white sugar
- 1 cup cream cheese
- 1 cup dried cranberries
- 1 teaspoon vanilla extract
- 2 teaspoons baking powder
- 3 cups all-purpose flour
- 4 eggs

Directions:
1. Mix the cranberries and Grand Marnier in a jar and allow to soak up for an hour.
2. Mix the flour with baking powder, baking soda and salt.
3. Mix the butter, cream cheese and sugar in a container until fluffy.
4. Stir in the eggs, one at a time, then put in the vanilla and milk.
5. Fold in the flour mixture and stir until incorporated.
6. Put in the cranberries.
7. Spoon the batter in a large loaf pan coated with baking paper.
8. Pre-heat the oven and bake at 350F for about fifty minutes or until a toothpick inserted in the center comes out clean.
9. Let the cake cool in the pan then serve, sliced.

Nutritional Content of One Serving:
Calories: 336 | Fat: 14.1g | Protein: 6.0g | Carbohydrates: 43.9g

Granny Smith Cake

Total Time Taken: 1 ½ hours
Yield: 12 Servings
Ingredients:

- ¼ teaspoon salt
- 1 ½ cups all-purpose flour
- 1 cup canola oil
- 1 cup white sugar
- 1 cup whole milk
- 1 tablespoon lemon zest
- 1 teaspoon cinnamon powder
- 2 eggs
- 2 teaspoons baking powder
- 3 Granny Smith apples, peeled and diced

Directions:
1. Sift the flour, baking powder, salt and cinnamon in a container.
2. In a separate container, combine the canola oil, eggs and sugar until fluffy and pale. Put in the milk and lemon zest and mix thoroughly.
3. Fold in the flour then mix in the apples.
4. Spoon the batter in a 9-inch round cake pan coated with baking paper.
5. Pre-heat the oven and bake at 350F for around forty minutes or until a toothpick comes out clean after being inserted into the center of the cake.
6. Serve chilled.

Nutritional Content of One Serving:

Calories: 328 | Fat: 19.8g | Protein: 3.3g | Carbohydrates: 36.4g

Hazelnut Chocolate Cake

Total Time Taken: 1 hour
Yield: 10 Servings
Ingredients:

- ½ cup butter
- ½ teaspoon salt
- 1 cup ground hazelnuts
- 1 cup Nutella
- 6 eggs, separated
- 6 oz. dark chocolate chips

Directions:

1. Combine the chocolate chips and butter in a heatproof container and place over a hot water bath.
2. Melt them together until smooth then turn off heat and fold in the egg yolks, followed by the Nutella and ground hazelnuts.
3. Whip the egg whites with a pinch of salt until firm then fold them in the batter using a spatula.
4. Pour the batter in a 9-inch round cake pan coated with baking paper.
5. Pre-heat the oven and bake at 350F for about half an hour.
6. Let the cake cool in the pan and serve, sliced.

Nutritional Content of One Serving:
Calories: 326 | Fat: 25.3g | Protein: 6.5g | Carbohydrates: 22.0g

Healthier Carrot Cake

Total Time Taken: 1 ½ hours
Yield: 10 Servings
Ingredients:

- ¼ cup orange juice
- ½ cup coconut oil, melted
- ½ cup grated apples
- ½ cup quinoa powder
- ½ cup raisins
- ½ cup rolled oats
- ½ teaspoon ground ginger
- ½ teaspoon salt
- 1 ½ cups grated carrots
- 1 cup low-fat yogurt cake
- 1 cup whole wheat flour
- 1 tablespoon orange zest
- 1 teaspoon cinnamon powder
- 2 teaspoons baking powder

Directions:

1. Mix the yogurt, orange juice, coconut oil, orange zest, carrots, apples and raisins.
2. Fold in the remaining ingredients and mix using a spatula.
3. Pour the batter in a 9-inch round cake pan coated with baking paper.
4. Pre-heat the oven and bake at 350F for about fifty minutes or until a toothpick inserted into the center of the cake comes out clean.
5. The cake tastes best chilled.

Nutritional Content of One Serving:
Calories: 215 | Fat: 12.0g | Protein: 2.9g | Carbohydrates: 25.1g

Holiday Pound Cake

Total Time Taken: 1 ¼ hours
Yield: 16 Servings
Ingredients:

- ½ teaspoon salt
- 1 cup butter, softened
- 1 cup buttermilk
- 1 cup cream cheese
- 1 teaspoon lemon zest
- 1 teaspoon orange zest
- 1 teaspoon vanilla extract
- 2 cups white sugar
- 2 teaspoons baking powder
- 3 cups all-purpose flour
- 6 eggs

Directions:

1. Mix the butter and sugar in a container until pale and light. Stir in the cream cheese and mix thoroughly.
2. Put in the eggs, one after another, then mix in the flour, baking powder and salt, alternating it with buttermilk.
3. Fold in the citrus zest and vanilla extract then spoon the batter in a large loaf cake pan coated with baking paper.
4. Preheat your oven and bake the cake for about fifty minutes or until a toothpick inserted into the center of the cake comes out clean.
5. Let the cake cool in the pan and serve, sliced.

Nutritional Content of One Serving:
Calories: 363 | Fat: 18.6g | Protein: 6.2g | Carbohydrates: 44.5g

Honey Fig Cake

Total Time Taken: 1 hour
Yield: 8 Servings
Ingredients:

- ½ cup butter, softened
- ½ cup honey
- ½ teaspoon salt
- 1 ½ cups all-purpose flour
- 1 teaspoon baking powder
- 1 teaspoon orange zest
- 1 teaspoon vanilla extract
- 1 whole egg
- 3 egg whites
- 6 fresh figs, quartered

Directions:

1. Mix the butter, honey, egg whites and egg in a container until creamy. Put in the vanilla and orange zest and mix thoroughly.
2. Fold in the flour, baking powder and salt then spoon the batter in a 9-inch round cake pan coated with baking paper.
3. Top the batter with fig slices and preheat your oven and bake at 350F for about forty minutes.
4. Let the cake cool in the pan and serve, sliced.

Nutritional Content of One Serving:

Calories: 304 | Fat: 12.4g | Protein: 5.1g | Carbohydrates: 45.0g

Hot Chocolate Bundt Cake

Total Time Taken: 1 hour

Yield: 12 Servings

Ingredients:

Cake:

- ½ cup canola oil
- ½ teaspoon salt
- ¾ cup butter, softened
- ¾ cup cocoa powder
- 1 cup hot water
- 1 cup light brown sugar
- 1 teaspoon vanilla extract
- 2 cups all-purpose flour
- 2 teaspoons baking powder
- 3 eggs
- 4 oz. dark chocolate, melted

Glaze:

- ½ cup heavy cream
- 1 cup dark chocolate chips

Directions:

1. For the cake, combine the butter, oil and sugar in a container until creamy and light.
2. Stir in the eggs, vanilla and melted chocolate.
3. Sift the flour with cocoa powder, baking powder and salt and fold it in the butter mixture.
4. Progressively mix in the hot water then spoon the batter in a greased Bundt cake pan.
5. Pre-heat the oven and bake at 350F for about forty minutes or until a toothpick inserted into the center of the cake comes out clean.
6. When finished, take out of the pan on a platter.
7. For the glaze, bring the cream to the boiling point then mix in the chocolate. Stir until melted and smooth.
8. Sprinkle the glaze over the cake and serve chilled.

Nutritional Content of One Serving:

Calories: 448 | Fat: 29.9g | Protein: 6.1g | Carbohydrates: 43.6g

Jam Studded Cake

Total Time Taken: 1 hour

Yield: 8 Servings

Ingredients: 5 eggs

- ¼ cup canola oil
- ¼ teaspoon salt
- ¾ cup white sugar
- 1 cup all-purpose flour
- 1 cup apricot jam
- 1 teaspoon baking powder
- 1 teaspoon orange zest
- 1 teaspoon vanilla extract

Directions:

1. Mix the eggs and sugar in a container until its volume increases to almost three times it was.
2. Stir in the oil, vanilla and orange zest then fold in the flour, baking powder and salt.
3. Spoon the batter in 1 9-inch round cake pan coated with baking paper.
4. Drop spoonfuls of apricot jam over the batter and preheat your oven and bake at 350F for around forty minutes or until a golden-brown colour is achieved and it rises significantly.
5. Let the cake cool in the pan and serve, sliced.

Nutritional Content of One Serving:

Calories: 326 | Fat: 9.8g | Protein: 5.4g | Carbohydrates: 57.1g

Lemon Blueberry Bundt Cake

Total Time Taken: 1 ¼ hours

Yield: 10 Servings

Ingredients:

- ½ cup butter, softened
- ½ cup cream cheese
- ½ teaspoon salt
- 1 ½ teaspoons baking powder
- 1 cup fresh blueberries
- 1 cup plain yogurt
- 1 cup white sugar
- 1 tablespoon lemon zest
- 1 teaspoon vanilla extract
- 2 cups all-purpose flour
- 2 egg whites
- 2 eggs

Directions:

1. Mix the butter, cream cheese and sugar in a container until creamy.
2. Stir in the eggs, egg whites, lemon zest and vanilla.
3. Fold in the flour, baking powder and salt, alternating it with yogurt.
4. Put in the blueberries then spoon the batter in a greased Bundt cake pan.

5. Pre-heat the oven and bake at 350F for about forty minutes or until a toothpick inserted in the center comes out clean.
6. Let the cake cool in the pan and serve, sliced.

Nutritional Content of One Serving:
Calories: 332 | Fat: 14.7g | Protein: 6.9g | Carbohydrates: 43.9g

Lemon Ginger Cake

Total Time Taken: 1 ¼ hours
Yield: 10 Servings
Ingredients:

- ¼ cup lemon juice
- ¼ teaspoon salt
- ½ teaspoon baking powder
- 1 ½ cups white sugar
- 1 cup butter, softened
- 1 cup sour cream
- 1 tablespoon lemon zest
- 1 teaspoon baking soda
- 1 teaspoon grated ginger
- 2 ½ cups all-purpose flour
- 4 eggs

Directions:

1. Sift the flour, baking soda, baking powder and salt.
2. Mix the butter and sugar in a container until creamy and fluffy.
3. Put in the eggs, one at a time, then mix in the lemon juice, lemon zest and ginger, as well as the sour cream.
4. Fold in the sifted flour then spoon the batter in a 9-inch round cake pan coated with baking paper.
5. Pre-heat the oven and bake at 350F for around forty minutes or until a toothpick comes out clean after being inserted into the center of the cake.
6. Let the cake cool in the pan and serve, sliced.

Nutritional Content of One Serving:
Calories: 466 | Fat: 25.4g | Protein: 6.4g | Carbohydrates: 55.5g

Lemon Raspberry Pound Cake

Total Time Taken: 1 ¼ hours
Yield: 10 Servings
Ingredients:
Cake:

- ½ cup cream cheese
- ½ teaspoon salt
- 1 ½ cups fresh raspberries
- 1 cup butter, softened
- 1 cup white sugar
- 1 teaspoon baking powder
- 1 teaspoon baking soda
- 1 teaspoon lemon zest
- 1 teaspoon vanilla extract
- 2 ¼ cups all-purpose flour
- 2 tablespoons lemon juice
- 4 eggs

Glaze:

- ½ cup cream cheese
- 1 teaspoon lemon zest
- 2 tablespoons lemon juice
- 2 tablespoons powdered sugar

Directions:

1. For the cake, sift the flour, baking soda, baking powder and salt in a container.
2. In a separate container, combine the butter, cream cheese, sugar, vanilla and lemon zest until creamy.
3. Stir in the eggs, one at a time, then put in the lemon juice.
4. Fold in the flour, mixing using a spatula.
5. Put in the raspberries then spoon the batter in a loaf cake pan coated with baking paper.
6. Pre-heat the oven and bake at 350F for about forty minutes or until a toothpick inserted into the center of the cake comes out clean.
7. When the cake is finished cooking, move it to a platter.
8. For the glaze, combine all the ingredients in a container.
9. Sprinkle the glaze over the cake and serve it fresh.

Nutritional Content of One Serving:
Calories: 466 | Fat: 28.7g | Protein: 7.3g | Carbohydrates: 46.5g

Lemon Ricotta Cake

Total Time Taken: 1 hour
Yield: 8 Servings
Ingredients:

- ¼ cup butter, melted
- ¼ teaspoon salt
- ½ cup almond flour
- ¾ cup white sugar
- 1 ¼ cups all-purpose flour
- 1 cup ricotta cheese
- 1 teaspoon baking powder
- 2 eggs
- 2 tablespoons lemon zest

Directions:

1. Mix the cheese, eggs, sugar, butter and lemon zest in a container.
2. Fold in the flours, baking powder and salt then spoon the batter in a 8-inch round cake pan coated with baking paper.
3. Pre-heat the oven and bake at 350F for around forty minutes or until a toothpick comes out clean after being inserted into the center of the cake.

4. *The cake tastes best chilled.*

Nutritional Content of One Serving:

Calories: 262 | Fat: 10.4g | Protein: 7.4g | Carbohydrates: 36.3g

Lemon Sprinkle Cake

Total Time Taken: 1 ¼ hours

Yield: 10 Servings

Ingredients:

Cake:

- ½ cup butter, melted
- ½ cup sour cream
- 1 ½ cups all-purpose flour
- 1 cup white sugar
- 1 teaspoon baking powder
- 2 tablespoons lemon juice
- 2 tablespoons lemon zest
- 5 eggs

Icing:

- 1 cup powdered sugar
- 1 tablespoon lemon juice
- 1 teaspoon lemon zest

Directions:

1. For the cake, combine the eggs and sugar in a container until twofold in volume and fluffy.
2. Put in the melted butter and stir lightly. Stir in the sour cream, lemon zest and lemon juice.
3. Fold in the flour, baking powder and salt then pour the batter in a 9-inch round cake pan covered with parchment paper.
4. Pre-heat the oven and bake at 350F for around forty minutes or until a golden-brown colour is achieved and it rises significantly.
5. Let the cake cool in the pan then move to a platter.
6. For the icing, combine all the ingredients then sprinkle it over the cake.
7. *Serve immediately.*

Nutritional Content of One Serving:

Calories: 330 | Fat: 14.0g | Protein: 5.2g | Carbohydrates: 47.5g

Lime Pound Cake

Total Time Taken: 1 ¼ hours

Yield: 12 Servings

Ingredients:

- ¼ cup canola oil
- ½ cup sour cream
- ½ teaspoon salt
- 1 ½ cups white sugar
- 1 cup butter, softened
- 1 lime, zested and juiced
- 1 teaspoon baking soda
- 2 cups all-purpose flour
- 4 eggs

Directions:

1. Mix the butter, oil and sugar in a container until pale and creamy.
2. Stir in the eggs and mix thoroughly then put in the lime zest and lime juice. Stir thoroughly to mix.
3. Fold in the dry ingredients then put in the sour cream.
4. Pulse using a mixer on high speed for a minute.
5. Spoon the batter in a loaf cake pan and preheat your oven and bake at 350F for about forty minutes or until it rises significantly and starts to appear golden-brown.
6. Let the cake cool in the pan and serve, sliced.

Nutritional Content of One Serving:

Calories: 389 | Fat: 23.6g | Protein: 4.5g | Carbohydrates: 42.0g

Madeira Cake

Total Time Taken: 1 hour

Yield: 8 Servings

Ingredients:

- ¼ cup whole milk
- ¼ teaspoon salt
- ¾ cup butter, softened
- ¾ cup white sugar
- 3 eggs
- 1 ½ cups all-purpose flour
- 1 teaspoon baking powder
- 1 teaspoon lemon zest

Directions:

1. Mix the butter and sugar in a container until creamy and firm. Put in the eggs, one at a time, then fold in the flour, baking powder and salt, alternating it with milk.
2. Put in the lemon zest then spoon the batter in a 9-inch round cake pan coated with baking paper.
3. Preheat your oven and bake the cake for around forty minutes or until it rises significantly and starts to appear golden-brown.
4. Let the cake cool in the pan and serve, sliced.

Nutritional Content of One Serving:

Calories: 337 | Fat: 19.4g | Protein: 4.9g | Carbohydrates: 37.5g

Mango Ice Box Cake

Total Time Taken: 1 hour

Yield: 8 Servings

Ingredients:

- ½ cup white sugar
- 1 tablespoon lemon juice
- 1/3 cup sweetened condensed milk
- 15 graham crackers
- 2 cups heavy cream, whipped
- 2 ripe mangos, peeled and cubed

Directions:

1. Mix the mangos, sugar and lemon juice in a saucepan and place over low heat. Cook for about ten minutes until softened. Let cool completely.
2. To finish the cake, take a loaf pan and line it using plastic wrap.
3. Mix the cream and sweetened condensed milk.
4. Layer the crackers with the mango mixture and cream in the readied pan.
5. Wrap securely and store in the refrigerator for minimum an hour.
6. *The cake tastes best chilled.*

Nutritional Content of One Serving:

Calories: 303 | Fat: 14.9g | Protein: 3.5g | Carbohydrates: 40.5g

Maple Syrup Apple Cake

Total Time Taken: 1 ¼ hours

Yield: 10 Servings

Ingredients:

- ¼ cup butter, softened
- ½ cup walnuts, chopped
- ½ cup whole milk
- ½ teaspoon salt
- 1 cup maple syrup
- 1 teaspoon cinnamon powder
- 1 teaspoon ground ginger
- 2 cups all-purpose flour
- 2 red apples, peeled, cored and diced
- 2 teaspoons baking powder
- 4 eggs

Directions:

1. Mix the flour, baking powder, cinnamon, ginger and salt in a container.
1. In a separate container, combine the butter and maple syrup. Stir in the eggs and the milk then fold in the flour.
2. Put in the apples and walnuts then spoon the batter in a Bundt cake pan lined using butter.
3. Pre-heat the oven and bake at 350F for around forty minutes or until it rises significantly and starts to appear golden-brown.
4. Let the cake cool in the pan and serve, sliced.

Nutritional Content of One Serving:

Calories: 306 | Fat: 10.8g | Protein: 6.8g | Carbohydrates: 47.1g

Marble Cake

Total Time Taken: 1 hour

Yield: 10 Servings

Ingredients:

- ¼ cup cocoa powder
- ¼ cup hot water
- ½ cup butter, softened
- ½ teaspoon baking soda
- ½ teaspoon salt
- 1 cup white sugar
- 1 cup whole milk
- 1 teaspoon vanilla extract
- 2 ½ cups all-purpose flour
- 2 teaspoon baking powder
- 3 eggs

Directions:

1. Mix the cocoa powder with hot water in a small container.
2. Mix the butter and sugar in a container until creamy and firm. Put in the eggs, one at a time, then mix in the vanilla and milk.
3. Fold in the flour, baking powder, baking soda and salt.
4. Divide the batter in half. Spoon one half in a loaf pan coated with baking paper.
5. Mix the half that is left over of batter with the cocoa mixture.
6. Spoon the cocoa batter over the white one and swirl it around with a toothpick.
7. Preheat your oven and bake the cake at 350F for around forty minutes or until a toothpick inserted in the center comes out clean.
8. Let the cake cool in the pan and serve, sliced.

Nutritional Content of One Serving:

Calories: 311 | Fat: 11.9g | Protein: 6.2g | Carbohydrates: 46.8g

Matcha Chocolate Cake

Total Time Taken: 1 ¼ hours

Yield: 8 Servings

Ingredients:

Cake:

- ¼ cup butter, melted
- ½ teaspoon salt
- 1 ¼ cups all-purpose flour
- 1 ½ teaspoons matcha powder
- 1 cup white sugar
- 1 teaspoon baking powder Chocolate
- 4 eggs
- 4 tablespoons hot water

Glaze:

- ¼ cup butter
- 1 cup dark chocolate chips

Directions:

1. For the cake, sift the flour with salt, matcha powder and baking powder.
2. Mix the eggs and white sugar until volume increases to twice what it was.
3. Stir in the melted butter and hot water then fold in the flour mixture.
4. Spoon the batter in a 9-inch round cake pan coated with baking paper.

5. Preheat your oven and bake the cake for around forty minutes or until a toothpick inserted in the center comes out clean.
6. For the glaze, mix the chocolate chips and butter in a heatproof container and place over a hot water bath. Melt them together until the desired smoothness is achieved.
7. Sprinkle the glaze over the cake and serve immediately or place in your refrigerator.

Nutritional Content of One Serving:
Calories: 371 | Fat: 17.9g | Protein: 5.9g | Carbohydrates: 51.0g

Matcha Pound Cake

Total Time Taken: 1 hour
Yield: 10 Servings
Ingredients:

- ¼ teaspoon salt
- ½ cup butter, softened
- ½ cup light brown sugar
- 1 cup all-purpose flour
- 1 tablespoon lemon juice
- 1 teaspoon baking powder
- 1 teaspoon lemon zest
- 2 teaspoons matcha powder
- 4 eggs, separated

Directions:

1. Sift the flour, salt, baking powder and matcha powder in a container.
2. Mix the butter with sugar until creamy and pale. Stir in the egg yolks and mix thoroughly. Put in the lemon zest and lemon juice and give it a good mix.
3. Fold in the flour.
4. Whip the egg whites until fluffy and firm. Fold the meringue into the cake batter.
5. Pour the batter in a loaf cake pan coated with baking paper.
6. Pre-heat the oven and bake at 350F for about forty minutes or until a toothpick inserted into the center of the cake comes out clean.
7. *The cake tastes best chilled.*

Nutritional Content of One Serving:
Calories: 185 | Fat: 11.1g | Protein: 3.6g | Carbohydrates: 18.1g

Meringue Black Forest Cake

Total Time Taken: 2 ½ hours
Yield: 8 Servings
Ingredients:

- ¼ teaspoon salt
- ½ teaspoon cream of tartar
- 1 ½ cups dark chocolate chips
- 1 cup heavy cream
- 1 cup sour cherries, pitted
- 1 cup white sugar
- 1 teaspoon vanilla extract
- 2 tablespoons cocoa powder
- 4 egg whites

Directions:

1. Mix the egg whites, cream of tartar and salt in a container for minimum five minutes or until firm and fluffy.
2. Put in the sugar, progressively, whipping until shiny and firm.
3. Fold in the cocoa powder then spoon the meringue on a large baking sheet coated with baking paper, shaping it into two 8-inch rounds.
4. Pre-heat the oven and bake at 250F for about two hours.
5. Bring the cream to the boiling point in a saucepan. Put in the chocolate and stir until it melts completely. Allow this cream to cool down then put in the vanilla.
6. Layer the baked meringue with chocolate cream and sour cherries.
7. *Serve the cake fresh.*

Nutritional Content of One Serving:
Calories: 275 | Fat: 11.8g | Protein: 3.9g | Carbohydrates: 44.1g

Milk Chocolate Chunk Cake

Total Time Taken: 1 1/5 hours
Yield: 12 Servings
Ingredients:

- ½ cup chocolate syrup
- ½ cup cocoa powder
- ½ teaspoon baking soda
- ½ teaspoon salt
- 1 cup butter, softened
- 1 cup buttermilk
- 1 cup white sugar
- 1 teaspoon baking powder
- 1 teaspoon vanilla extract
- 2 cups all-purpose flour
- 4 eggs
- 8 oz. milk chocolate, chopped

Directions:

1. Sift the flour, cocoa powder, baking powder, baking soda and salt.
2. Mix the butter with sugar until creamy and fluffy. Put in the chocolate syrup then mix in the eggs and vanilla.
3. Fold in the flour, alternating it with buttermilk. Begin and finish with flour.
4. Put in the chocolate chunks then spoon the batter in a round cake pan coated with baking paper.
5. Pre-heat the oven and bake at 350F for about forty minutes or until a toothpick comes out clean after being inserted into the center of the cake.

Nutritional Content of One Serving:
Calories: 449 | Fat: 23.4g | Protein: 7.2g | Carbohydrates: 55.2g

Mississippi Mud Cake

Total Time Taken: 1 ¼ hours
Yield: 12 Servings
Ingredients:

- ½ cup cocoa powder
- ½ teaspoon salt
- 1 cup buttermilk
- 1 cup canola oil
- 1 cup hot coffee
- 1 teaspoon baking powder
- 1 teaspoon baking soda
- 2 ½ cups all-purpose flour
- 2 cups white sugar
- 2 eggs
- 2 teaspoons vanilla extract

Directions:

1. Mix the sugar, eggs, coffee, oil, vanilla and buttermilk in a container.
2. In a separate container, mix the cocoa powder, salt, flour, baking soda and baking powder then mix in the coffee mixture.
3. Pour the batter in a 10-inch round cake pan covered with parchment paper.
4. Pre-heat the oven and bake at 330F for about fifty minutes.
5. Let the cake cool in the pan and serve, sliced.

Nutritional Content of One Serving:
Calories: 410 | Fat: 19.8g | Protein: 5.0g | Carbohydrates: 56.5g

Moist Apple Cake

Total Time Taken: 1 ½ hours
Yield: 14 Servings
Ingredients:

- ¼ cup maple syrup
- ½ teaspoon salt
- 1 ½ cups light brown sugar
- 1 cup butter, softened
- 1 teaspoon cinnamon powder
- 1 teaspoon ground cardamom
- 1 teaspoon ground ginger
- 2 cups applesauce
- 2 eggs
- 2 green apples, peeled, cored and diced
- 2 teaspoons baking soda
- 3 cups all-purpose flour

Directions:

1. Mix the flour, baking soda, salt and spices in a container.
2. In a separate container, mix the butter, sugar and maple syrup and stir thoroughly for a few minutes.
3. Stir in the eggs and applesauce then fold in the flour mixture.
4. Put in the apples then spoon the batter in a 10-inch round cake pan coated with baking paper.
5. Pre-heat the oven and bake at 350F for about fifty minutes or until a toothpick inserted into the center of the cake comes out clean.
6. Let the cake cool in the pan and serve, sliced.

Nutritional Content of One Serving:
Calories: 326 | Fat: 14.1g | Protein: 3.9g | Carbohydrates: 47.2g

Moist Chocolate Cake

Total Time Taken: 1 ¼ hours
Yield: 12 Servings
Ingredients:

- ½ cup canola oil
- ½ cup cocoa powder
- ½ teaspoon salt
- 1 ½ teaspoon baking powder
- 1 cup buttermilk
- 1 cup hot coffee
- 1 teaspoon vanilla extract
- 2 cups all-purpose flour
- 2 cups white sugar
- 2 eggs

Directions:

1. Mix the sugar, eggs and canola oil in a container until creamy.
2. Stir in the vanilla, coffee and buttermilk then put in the remaining ingredients.
3. Pour the batter in a 9-inch round cake pan coated with baking paper.
4. Pre-heat the oven and bake at 350F for about forty-five minutes or until a toothpick comes out clean after being inserted into the center of the cake.
5. Let the cake cool in the pan before you serve.

Nutritional Content of One Serving:
Calories: 310 | Fat: 10.7g | Protein: 4.4g | Carbohydrates: 52.6g

Moist Pumpkin Cake

Total Time Taken: 1 ¼ hours
Yield: 12 Servings
Ingredients:

- ¼ teaspoon ground nutmeg
- ½ teaspoon ground ginger
- ½ teaspoon salt
- 1 ½ cups pumpkin puree
- 1 cup canola oil
- 1 teaspoon cinnamon powder
- 2 cups white sugar
- 2 teaspoons baking powder
- 3 cups all-purpose flour
- 4 eggs

Directions:

1. Mix the sugar, canola oil and eggs in a container until creamy and volume increases to twice what it was.
2. Stir in the pumpkin puree, then fold in the remaining ingredients.
3. Pour the batter in a 9-inch round cake pan coated with baking paper.
4. Pre-heat the oven and bake at 350F for around forty minutes or until well risen and fragrant.
5. Let the cake cool in the pan and serve, sliced.

Nutritional Content of One Serving:
Calories: 432 | Fat: 20.1g | Protein: 5.4g | Carbohydrates: 60.2g

Molasses Pear Bundt Cake

Total Time Taken: 1 ¼ hours
Yield: 10 Servings
Ingredients:

- ½ cup light brown sugar
- ½ cup molasses
- ½ cup sour cream
- ½ cup whole milk
- ½ teaspoon ground ginger
- ½ teaspoon salt
- 1 cup butter, softened
- 1 teaspoon all-spice
- 1 teaspoon baking powder
- 1 teaspoon baking soda
- 1 teaspoon cinnamon powder
- 2 cups all-purpose flour
- 2 pears, peeled, cored and diced
- 3 eggs

Directions:

1. Mix the butter, molasses and sugar in a container until creamy and pale.
2. Stir in the eggs, one at a time, stirring thoroughly after each addition.
3. Mix the flour with baking powder, baking soda, salt and spices.
4. Mix the milk with cream.
5. Fold the flour into the butter mixture, alternating it with the milk and sour cream mix.
6. Put in the pears then spoon the batter in a greased Bundt cake pan.
7. Pre-heat the oven and bake at 350F for about forty minutes or until a toothpick inserted in the center comes out clean.
8. Let the cake cool in the pan for about ten minutes then flip over on a platter.
9. Serve chilled.

Nutritional Content of One Serving:
Calories: 405 | Fat: 22.9g | Protein: 5.3g | Carbohydrates: 46.3g

Morello Cherry Cake

Total Time Taken: 1 ¼ hours
Yield: 12 Servings
Ingredients:

- ¼ cup brandy
- ½ cup cocoa powder
- ½ cup cocoa powder
- ½ cup coconut oil, melted
- ½ cup white sugar
- ½ teaspoon salt
- ¾ cup all-purpose flour
- 1 cup almond flour
- 1 cup maple syrup
- 1 cup Morello cherries
- 3 eggs

Directions:

1. Mix the maple syrup, coconut oil, brandy and eggs in a container.
2. Stir in the sugar and mix thoroughly.
3. Fold in the cocoa powder, almond flour, all-purpose flour, salt and cocoa powder.
4. Spoon the batter in a 9-inch round cake pan and top with cherries.
5. Pre-heat the oven and bake at 350F for forty minutes.
6. *The cake tastes best chilled.*

Nutritional Content of One Serving:
Calories: 270 | Fat: 12.4g | Protein: 4.2g | Carbohydrates: 40.9g

Natural Red Velvet Cake

Total Time Taken: 1 ¼ hours
Yield: 10 Servings
Ingredients:
Cake:

- ¼ cup white sugar
- ½ cup canola oil
- ½ cup light brown sugar
- ½ teaspoon cinnamon powder
- ½ teaspoon salt
- 1 ¼ cups all-purpose flour
- 1 teaspoon baking powder
- 2 beetroots, peeled and pureed
- 2 eggs
- 2 tablespoons cornstarch

Frosting:

- ¼ cup butter, softened
- 1 cup cream cheese
- 1 cup powdered sugar

Directions:

1. For the cake, combine the beetroot puree, canola oil, eggs and sugar in a container.
2. Stir in the remaining ingredients and mix thoroughly.
3. Pour the batter in a 8-inch round cake pan coated with baking paper.

4. Pre-heat the oven and bake at 350F for forty minutes.
5. When finished, allow the cake to cool in the pan then transfer the cake on a platter.
6. For the frosting, combine all the ingredients in a container until fluffy.
7. Cover the cake with the frosting and serve it fresh.

Nutritional Content of One Serving:
Calories: 395 | Fat: 24.7g | Protein: 4.8g | Carbohydrates: 40.1g

Olive Oil Pistachio Cake

Total Time Taken: 1 hour
Yield: 10 Servings
Ingredients:

- ½ cup corn meal
- ½ cup extra virgin olive oil
- ½ cup ground pistachios
- ½ cup white sugar
- 3 eggs
- ½ cup whole milk
- ½ teaspoon salt
- 1 cup all-purpose flour
- 1 teaspoon baking powder
- 1 teaspoon baking soda
- 2 tablespoons orange zest

Directions:
1. Mix the dry ingredients in a container.
2. In a separate container, mix the oil, sugar, eggs and orange zest and stir thoroughly for a few minutes until volume increases to twice what it was.
3. Stir in the milk, followed by the dry ingredients.
4. Pour the batter in 10-inch round cake pan coated with baking paper.
5. Preheat your oven and bake the cake for around forty minutes.
6. The cake tastes best chilled.

Nutritional Content of One Serving:
Calories: 221 | Fat: 12.1g | Protein: 4.0g | Carbohydrates: 26.1g

Orange Chocolate Cake

Total Time Taken: 1 ¼ hours
Yield: 12 Servings
Ingredients:

- ½ cup candied orange peel, chopped
- ½ teaspoon salt
- 1 cup white sugar
- 1 teaspoon baking soda
- 2 cups ground almonds
- 4 eggs
- 8 oz. dark chocolate, melted

Directions:
1. Mix the eggs with sugar until fluffy and pale.
2. Stir in the melted chocolate then put in the almonds, baking soda and salt.
3. Fold in the candied orange peel then pour the batter in 1 8-inch round cake pan coated with baking paper.
4. Pre-heat the oven and bake at 350F for about half an hour.
5. Let the cake cool in the pan before you serve.

Nutritional Content of One Serving:
Calories: 280 | Fat: 15.0g | Protein: 6.7g | Carbohydrates: 32.4g

Orange Chocolate Mud Cake

Total Time Taken: 1 ¼ hours
Yield: 10 Servings
Ingredients:

- ½ cup brewed coffee
- ½ cup candied orange peel, chopped
- ½ teaspoon salt
- ¾ cup cocoa powder
- 1 ½ cups all-purpose flour
- 1 cup butter, softened
- 1 tablespoon orange zest
- 1 teaspoon baking soda
- 1 teaspoon vanilla extract
- 2 cups white sugar
- 2 tablespoons cornstarch
- 4 eggs

Directions:
1. Mix the sugar and butter in a container until fluffy and pale.
2. Put in the coffee, eggs, vanilla and orange zest.
3. Stir in the remaining ingredients and mix thoroughly.
4. Pour the batter in a 9-inch round cake pan coated with baking paper.
5. Preheat your oven and bake the cake for about fifty minutes or until the cake looks set.
6. *The cake tastes best chilled.*

Nutritional Content of One Serving:
Calories: 433 | Fat: 21.2g | Protein: 5.6g | Carbohydrates: 60.9g

Orange Pound Cake

Total Time Taken: 1 ¼ hours
Yield: 16 Servings
Ingredients:

- ½ teaspoon salt
- 1 ½ cups butter, softened
- 1 cup sour cream
- 1 orange, zested and juiced
- 1 teaspoon vanilla extract
- 2 cups white sugar
- 2 teaspoons baking powder

- 3 cups all-purpose flour
- 6 eggs

Directions:

1. Sift the flour with salt and baking powder.
2. Mix the butter with sugar for five minutes until creamy and fluffy.
3. Put in the vanilla, orange zest and orange juice and mix thoroughly.
4. Stir in the sour cream then fold in the flour mixture.
5. Pour the batter in a large loaf cake pan coated with baking paper.
6. Pre-heat the oven and bake at 330F for forty minutes then turn the heat on 350F for another ten minutes.
7. Let the cake cool in the pan and serve, sliced.

Nutritional Content of One Serving:
Calories: 393 | Fat: 22.2g | Protein: 5.2g | Carbohydrates: 45.3g

Orange Pumpkin Bundt Cake

Total Time Taken: 1 ¼ hours
Yield: 12 Servings
Ingredients:

- ½ teaspoon cinnamon powder
- ½ teaspoon ground cardamom
- ½ teaspoon ground ginger
- ½ teaspoon salt
- ¾ cup butter, softened
- 1 ¼ cups white sugar
- 1 ½ teaspoons baking soda
- 1 cup pumpkin puree
- 1 orange, zested and juiced
- 1 teaspoon vanilla extract
- 2 ½ cups all-purpose flour
- 4 eggs

Directions:

1. Mix the butter with sugar in a container until creamy and fluffy.
2. Stir in the eggs and vanilla and mix thoroughly then put in the orange zest and juice, as well as pumpkin puree.
3. Fold in the rest of the ingredients then spoon the batter in a loaf cake pan coated with baking paper.
4. Preheat your oven and bake the cake for about forty minutes.
5. Let the cake cool in the pan before you serve.

Nutritional Content of One Serving:
Calories: 311 | Fat: 13.3g | Protein: 5.0g | Carbohydrates: 44.4g

Orange Ricotta Cake

Total Time Taken: 1 ¼ hours
Yield: 10 Servings
Ingredients:

- ½ cup all-purpose flour
- ½ cup white chocolate, chopped
- ¾ cup white sugar
- 1 cup fresh raspberries
- 1 teaspoon baking powder
- 1 teaspoon orange zest
- 1 teaspoon vanilla extract
- 3 cups ricotta cheese
- 3 eggs

Directions:

1. Mix the ricotta cheese, vanilla, orange zest, sugar and eggs in a container.
2. Stir in rest of the ingredients then spoon the batter in a 9-inch round cake pan coated with baking paper.
3. Pre-heat the oven and bake at 350F for around forty minutes or until a golden-brown colour is achieved.
4. The cake tastes best chilled.

Nutritional Content of One Serving:
Calories: 255 | Fat: 10.1g | Protein: 11.4g | Carbohydrates: 30.5g

Parsnip Carrot Cake

Total Time Taken: 1 ½ hours
Yield: 12 Servings
Ingredients:

- ¼ cup white sugar
- ½ cup walnuts, chopped
- ½ teaspoon salt
- 1 cup canola oil
- 1 cup crushed pineapple
- 1 cup grated carrots
- 1 cup grated parsnips
- 1 cup light brown sugar
- 1 teaspoon baking powder
- 1 teaspoon baking soda
- 1 teaspoon cinnamon powder
- 1 teaspoon ground ginger
- 2 cups all-purpose flour
- 4 eggs

Directions:

1. Mix the flour, salt, baking soda, baking powder and spices in a container.
2. In a separate container, combine the eggs with the sugars until fluffy and pale.
3. Put in the oil then mix in the carrots, parsnips, pineapple and walnuts.
4. Fold in the dry ingredients you readied a while back.
5. Pour the batter in a 9-inch round cake pan coated with baking paper.

6. Pre-heat the oven and bake at 350F for about forty minutes or until a toothpick inserted in the center comes out clean.
7. Sprinkle with powdered sugar and serve chilled.

Nutritional Content of One Serving:
Calories: 371 | Fat: 23.0g | Protein: 5.5g | Carbohydrates: 37.6g

Peach Brandy Cake

Total Time Taken: 1 ½ hours
Yield: 10 Servings
Ingredients:
Cake:

- ½ cup butter, melted
- ½ teaspoon salt
- 1 cup sweet red win
- 1 cup white sugar
- 1 teaspoon baking powder
- 1 teaspoon ground cardamom
- 2 cups almond flour
- 4 peaches, pitted and sliced Brandy
- 5 eggs

Glaze:

- 1 cup powdered sugar
- 1 tablespoon brandy

Directions:

1. To prepare the cake, combine the almond flour, baking powder, salt and cinnamon.
2. In a separate container, combine the sugar and eggs until fluffy and pale. Put in the butter and mix thoroughly, then mix in the red wine.
3. Fold in the almond flour then pour the batter in a 9-inch round cake pan coated with baking paper.
4. Top with sliced peaches and preheat your oven and bake at 350F for 45 minutes or until a toothpick comes out clean after being inserted into the center of the cake.
5. Let the cake cool in the pan then move it to a platter.
6. For the glaze, combine the sugar with brandy. Sprinkle the glaze over the cake and serve it fresh.

Nutritional Content of One Serving:
Calories: 317 | Fat: 15.8g | Protein: 8.3g | Carbohydrates: 37.4g

Peach Meringue Cake

Total Time Taken: 1 ½ hours
Yield: 10 Servings
Ingredients:
Cake:

- ½ cup butter, softened
- ½ cup canola oil
- ½ cup plain yogurt
- ½ teaspoon salt
- ¾ cup white sugar
- 1 teaspoon baking soda
- 1 teaspoon vanilla extract
- 2 cups all-purpose flour
- 3 eggs
- 3 peaches, pitted and sliced

Meringue:

- ½ cup white sugar
- 1 teaspoon vanilla extract
- 3 egg whites

Directions:

1. For the cake, combine the butter, oil and sugar in a container until fluffy and creamy.
2. Stir in the egg, vanilla and yogurt and mix thoroughly.
3. Fold in the flour, baking soda and salt then spoon the batter in a round cake pan coated with baking paper.
4. Top with peach slices and preheat your oven and bake at 350F for about forty minutes or until it rises significantly and starts to appear golden-brown.
5. While the cake bakes, combine the egg whites and sugar in a heatproof container.
6. Place over a hot water bath and mix with a whisk until the mixture is hot.
7. Turn off the heat and continue mixing until firm and shiny. Put in the vanilla and mix thoroughly.
8. Spoon the meringue over the hot cake and allow to cool.
9. *Serve immediately.*

Nutritional Content of One Serving:
Calories: 411 | Fat: 21.9g | Protein: 6.4g | Carbohydrates: 48.5g

Peach Upside Down Cake

Total Time Taken: 1 hour
Yield: 8 Servings
Ingredients:

- ¼ cup butter, melted
- ¼ cup whole milk
- ¼ teaspoon salt
- 1 egg
- ½ cup light brown sugar
- ½ cup sour cream
- 1 cup all-purpose flour
- 1 teaspoon baking powder
- 2 tablespoons butter
- 4 peaches, sliced

Directions:

1. Position the peaches at the bottom of a 9-inch round cake pan coated with baking paper.
2. Drizzle with brown sugar and top with a few pieces of butter.

3. For the batter, combine the flour, baking powder and salt in a container. Put in the rest of the ingredients and stir for a few seconds to mix.
4. Spoon the batter over the peaches and preheat your oven and bake at 350F for about half an hour.
5. When finished, flip the cake upside down on a platter.
6. Serve chilled.

Nutritional Content of One Serving:
Calories: 231 | Fat: 12.7g | Protein: 3.6g | Carbohydrates: 26.8g

Peanut Butter Chocolate Bundt Cake

Total Time Taken: 1 ¼ hours
Yield: 10 Servings
Ingredients:

- ¼ cup butter, softened
- ½ cup cocoa powder
- ½ cup dark chocolate chips
- ½ teaspoon baking soda
- ½ teaspoon salt
- 1 cup buttermilk
- 1 cup light brown sugar
- 1 cup smooth peanut butter
- 1 teaspoon vanilla extract
- 2 cups all-purpose flour
- 2 teaspoons baking powder
- 3 eggs

Directions:

1. Sift the flour, baking powder, baking soda, salt and cocoa powder.
2. Mix the peanut butter, butter and sugar in a container until creamy and light.
3. Put in the eggs and mix thoroughly then mix in the vanilla.
4. Fold in the flour, alternating it with buttermilk. Begin and finish with flour.
5. Put in the chocolate chips then spoon the batter in a Bundt cake pan lined using butter.
6. Preheat your oven and bake the cake for about forty minutes or until it rises significantly and starts to appear golden-brown.
7. When finished, flip the cake upside down on a platter and serve chilled.

Nutritional Content of One Serving:
Calories: 407 | Fat: 21.6g | Protein: 12.8g | Carbohydrates: 46.5g

Peanut Butter Jelly Cake

Total Time Taken: 1 ½ hours
Yield: 12 Servings
Ingredients:

- ½ cup butter, softened
- ½ cup cranberry jelly
- ½ cup light brown sugar
- ½ cup peanut butter
- ½ cup whole milk
- ½ teaspoon salt
- 1 cup white sugar
- 1 teaspoon vanilla extract
- 2 cups all-purpose flour
- 2 eggs
- 2 tablespoons canola oil
- 2 teaspoons baking powder

Directions:

1. Sift the flour, baking powder and salt.
2. Mix the peanut butter, butter, canola oil and sugars in a container until creamy and fluffy.
3. Stir in the eggs and vanilla and mix thoroughly.
4. Fold in the flour mixture, alternating it with the milk. Begin and finish with flour.
5. Spoon the batter in a round cake pan coated with baking paper.
6. Pre-heat the oven and bake at 350F for about forty minutes or until a toothpick inserted into the center of the cake comes out clean.
7. When finished, brush the cake with cranberry jelly and serve it fresh.

Nutritional Content of One Serving:
Calories: 334 | Fat: 16.7g | Protein: 6.2g | Carbohydrates: 42.0g

Pear Brownie Cake

Total Time Taken: 1 ¼ hours
Yield: 10 Servings
Ingredients:

- ¼ cup cocoa powder
- ¼ teaspoon salt
- ½ cup all-purpose flour
- ½ cup butter, softened
- ½ cup white sugar
- 1 cup dark chocolate chips
- 2 pears, peeled, cored and diced
- 4 eggs

Directions:

1. Mix the butter and chocolate in a heatproof container over a hot water bath. Melt them together until the desired smoothness is achieved.
2. Put in the eggs, one at a time, then mix in the sugar.
3. Fold in the flour, cocoa powder and salt then spoon the batter in a 8-inch round cake pan coated with baking paper.
4. Top with pear dices and preheat your oven and bake at 350F for 25 minutes.
5. Let the cake cool in the pan before you serve.

Nutritional Content of One Serving:
Calories: 252 | Fat: 14.6g | Protein: 4.3g | Carbohydrates: 30.5g

Pear Cinnamon Bundt Cake

Total Time Taken: 1 ¼ hours
Yield: 10 Servings
Ingredients:

- ½ cup buttermilk
- ½ teaspoon ground ginger
- ½ teaspoon salt
- 1 ½ cups light brown sugar
- 1 cup butter, melted
- 1 teaspoon cinnamon powder
- 2 cups all-purpose flour
- 2 pears, peeled, cored and diced
- 2 teaspoons baking powder
- 4 eggs

Directions:

1. Mix the flour, cinnamon, ginger, baking powder and salt in a container.
2. In a separate container, mix the butter, sugar, eggs and buttermilk and mix thoroughly. Pour this mixture over the dry ingredients then fold in the pears.
3. Spoon the batter in a Bundt cake pan lined using butter.
4. Pre-heat the oven and bake at 350F for around forty minutes or until golden and it rises significantly.
5. Let the cake cool in the pan before you serve.

Nutritional Content of One Serving:
Calories: 392 | Fat: 20.6g | Protein: 5.6g | Carbohydrates: 48.0g

Pecan Butter Cake

Total Time Taken: 1 ¼ hours
Yield: 12 Servings
Ingredients:

- ½ cup butter, softened
- ½ teaspoon salt
- 1 ½ cups pecans, chopped
- 1 ½ teaspoons baking powder
- 1 cup pecan butter
- 1 cup white sugar
- 1 teaspoon lemon zest
- 1 teaspoon vanilla extract
- 2 cups all-purpose flour
- 4 eggs

Directions:

1. Mix the two types of butter with sugar until creamy and light.
2. Stir in the eggs, one at a time, then put in the vanilla and lemon zest then fold in the dry ingredients.
3. Spoon the batter in a 9-inch round cake pan coated with baking paper.
4. Pre-heat the oven and bake at 350F for about forty minutes or until it rises significantly and starts to appear golden-brown.
5. Let the cake cool in the pan then sprinkle it with powdered sugar and serve.

Nutritional Content of One Serving:
Calories: 377 | Fat: 24.2g | Protein: 6.2g | Carbohydrates: 37.9g

Pecan Carrot Bundt Cake

Total Time Taken: 1 ½ hours
Yield: 14 Servings
Ingredients:

- ¼ cup orange juice
- ½ cup dark brown sugar
- ½ teaspoon baking powder
- ½ teaspoon cardamom powder
- ½ teaspoon salt
- 1 cup butter, softened
- 1 cup crushed pineapple
- 1 cup white sugar
- 1 tablespoon lemon zest
- 1 tablespoon orange zest
- 1 teaspoon baking soda
- 1 teaspoon cinnamon powder
- 2 ½ cups all-purpose flour
- 2 cups grated carrots
- 4 eggs

Directions:

1. Sift the flour, baking soda, baking powder, salt and spices in a container.
2. In a separate container, combine the butter and sugars until creamy and fluffy.
3. Stir in the eggs, one at a time, then put in the citrus zest, carrots, orange juice and pineapple.
4. Fold in the flour and stir lightly using a spatula.
5. Pour the batter in a greased Bundt cake pan.
6. Pre-heat the oven and bake at 350F for about fifty minutes or until a toothpick inserted into the center of the cake comes out clean.
7. Let the cake cool in the pan before you serve.

Nutritional Content of One Serving:
Calories: 304 | Fat: 14.6g | Protein: 4.3g | Carbohydrates: 40.4g

Pecan Rum Cake

Total Time Taken: 1 ¼ hours
Yield: 12 Servings
Ingredients:
Cake:

- ¼ cup dark rum
- ½ cup whole milk
- ½ teaspoon salt
- 1 ¼ cups all-purpose flour

- 1 cup butter, softened
- 1 cup ground pecans
- 1 cup white sugar
- 1 teaspoon baking soda
- 1 teaspoon vanilla extract
- 3 eggs

Glaze:

- 1 cup powdered sugar
- 1 tablespoon dark rum

Directions:

1. For the cake, combine the flour with baking soda, salt and pecans.
2. In a separate container, combine the butter and sugar until fluffy and creamy.
3. Stir in the eggs, one after another, then put in the vanilla, rum and milk and mix thoroughly.
4. Fold in the pecan and flour mixture then spoon the batter in a 8-inch round cake pan coated with baking paper.
5. Pre-heat the oven and bake at 350F for around forty minutes or until well risen and fragrant.
6. Let the cake cool in the pan then move to a platter.
7. For the glaze, combine the ingredients in a container. Sprinkle the glaze over the cake and serve fresh.

Nutritional Content of One Serving:

Calories: 329 | Fat: 17.8g | Protein: 3.3g | Carbohydrates: 37.3g

Peppermint Chocolate Cake

Total Time Taken: 1 ¼ hours

Yield: 10 Servings

Ingredients:

Cake:

- ½ cup canola oil
- 1 cup buttermilk
- ½ cup cocoa powder
- ½ cup hot coffee
- ½ teaspoon baking soda
- ½ teaspoon salt
- 1 ½ cups all-purpose flour
- 1 teaspoon baking powder
- 1 teaspoon vanilla extract

Frosting:

- ½ cup butter, softened
- 1 ½ cups powdered sugar
- 1 teaspoon peppermint extract
- 3 oz. dark chocolate, melted and cooled

Directions:

1. To prepare the cake, combine the dry ingredients in a container and the wet ingredients in a separate container.
2. Combine the flour mixture with the wet ingredients and stir for a few seconds to mix.
3. Pour the batter in a 9-inch cake pan coated with baking paper.
4. Pre-heat the oven and bake at 350F for about 35 minutes.
5. Let the cake cool in the pan then move to a platter.
6. For the frosting, combine the butter with the sugar until creamy and fluffy.
7. Put in the peppermint extract and the melted chocolate and mix thoroughly.
8. Frost the top of the cake with this chocolate buttercream and serve immediately or place in your refrigerator.

Nutritional Content of One Serving:

Calories: 384 | Fat: 23.6g | Protein: 4.3g | Carbohydrates: 41.2g

Pistachio Bundt Cake

Total Time Taken: 1 hour

Yield: 10 Servings

Ingredients:

- ½ teaspoon salt
- ¾ cup butter, softened
- 1 ½ cups all-purpose flour
- 1 ½ teaspoons baking powder
- 1 cup ground pistachio
- 1 cup white sugar
- 1 teaspoon vanilla extract
- 4 eggs

Directions:

1. Mix the butter and sugar until pale and light. Stir in the eggs and vanilla and mix thoroughly.
2. Fold in the flour, pistachio, baking powder and salt then spoon the batter in a greased Bundt cake pan.
3. Pre-heat the oven and bake at 350F for about forty minutes or until it rises significantly and starts to appear golden-brown.
4. Let the cake cool in the pan before you serve.

Nutritional Content of One Serving:

Calories: 292 | Fat: 15.7g | Protein: 4.3g | Carbohydrates: 34.9g

Pistachio Cake

Total Time Taken: 1 hour

Yield: 8 Servings

Ingredients:

- ¼ cup whole milk
- ¼ teaspoon cinnamon powder
- ¼ teaspoon salt
- ½ cup all-purpose flour
- ½ cup butter, softened
- ½ cup white sugar
- ½ teaspoon ground cardamom
- 1 cup ground pistachio

- 1 teaspoon baking powder
- 1 teaspoon lemon zest
- 2 eggs

Directions:

1. Mix the pistachio, flour, salt, baking powder, cardamom and cinnamon in a container.
2. Mix the butter and sugar in a container until fluffy and light. Stir in the eggs and milk, as well as lemon zest.
3. Fold in the flour and pistachio mixture then spoon the batter in a 8-inch round cake pan coated with baking paper.
4. Pre-heat the oven and bake at 350F for around forty minutes.
5. The cake tastes best chilled, dusted with powdered sugar.

Nutritional Content of One Serving:

Calories: 214 | Fat: 14.1g | Protein: 3.2g | Carbohydrates: 20.1g

Plum Polenta Cake

Total Time Taken: 1 hour

Yield: 8 Servings

Ingredients:

- ½ cup butter, softened
- ½ cup honey
- ½ pound plums, pitted and sliced
- ½ teaspoon salt
- ½ teaspoon salt
- 1 cup instant polenta flour
- 1 tablespoon lemon zest
- 1 teaspoon baking soda
- 2 cups whole milk
- 4 eggs

Directions:

1. Mix the butter with honey until creamy and firm. Stir in the eggs, one at a time, then put in the milk and lemon zest.
2. Fold in the polenta flour, baking soda and salt then pour the batter in a 9-inch round cake pan coated with baking paper.
3. Top with plum slices and preheat your oven and bake at 350F for around forty minutes or until a golden-brown colour is achieved and it rises significantly.
4. Let the cake cool in the pan then serve, sliced.

Nutritional Content of One Serving:

Calories: 298 | Fat: 15.7g | Protein: 7.1g | Carbohydrates: 33.7g

Pomegranate Cake

Total Time Taken: 1 ½ hours

Yield: 10 Servings

Ingredients:

White cake:

- ½ teaspoon salt
- ¾ cup whole milk
- 1 ¼ cups butter, softened
- 1 ½ cups all-purpose flour
- 1 ½ teaspoons baking powder
- 1 cup white sugar
- 1 teaspoon lemon zest
- 1 teaspoon vanilla extract
- 4 eggs whites

Pomegranate frosting:

- ¼ cup pomegranate juice
- 1 cup white sugar 1 pinch salt
- 4 egg whites

Directions:

1. Mix the flour with sugar, baking powder, salt and butter in a container until grainy.
2. Combine the egg whites with milk, vanilla and lemon zest in a container then pour this mixture over the flour mixture.
3. Stir slowly until mixed then spoon the batter into two 7-inch circular cake pans coated with baking paper.
4. Pre-heat the oven and bake at 350F for about half an hour.
5. Let the cakes cool in the pan then level them and cut each cake in half along the length.
6. For the frosting, combine all the ingredients in a heatproof container and place over a hot water bath. Keep over heat, stirring constantly, until the mixture is hot.
7. Turn off the heat and whip using an electric mixer for minimum seven minutes until firm and shiny.
8. Use half of the frosting to fill the cake and the rest of the frosting to frost the cake.
9. Serve immediately or place in your refrigerator.

Nutritional Content of One Serving:

Calories: 449 | Fat: 23.8g | Protein: 5.7g | Carbohydrates: 55.8g

Poppy Seed Lemon Bundt Cake

Total Time Taken: 1 ¼ hours

Yield: 12 Servings

Ingredients:

- ½ cup cornstarch
- ½ cup sour cream
- ½ teaspoon salt
- 1 cup butter, softened
- 1 cup white sugar
- 1 tablespoon lemon zest
- 1 teaspoon baking powder
- 1 teaspoon baking soda
- 1 teaspoon vanilla extract
- 2 cups all-purpose flour
- 2 tablespoons lemon juice

- 2 tablespoons poppy seeds
- 4 eggs

Directions:

1. Sift the flour, cornstarch, baking powder, baking soda and salt then mix it with the poppy seeds.
2. Mix the butter and sugar in a container until creamy and fluffy.
3. Stir in the eggs, lemon zest and lemon juice and mix thoroughly.
4. Fold in the flour mixture then put in the sour cream and mix thoroughly.
5. Spoon the batter in a greased Bundt cake pan and preheat your oven and bake at 350F for about forty minutes or until a toothpick comes out clean after being inserted into the center of the cake.
6. Let the cake cool in the pan before you serve.

Nutritional Content of One Serving:

Calories: 346 | Fat: 19.7g | Protein: 4.8g | Carbohydrates: 38.7g

Rainbow Cake

Total Time Taken: 1 hour

Yield: 10 Servings

Ingredients:

- ½ cup sour cream
- ½ teaspoon baking soda
- ½ teaspoon salt
- 1 ½ cups white sugar
- 1 cup butter, softened
- 1 teaspoon baking powder
- 1 teaspoon vanilla extract
- 2 ½ cups all-purpose flour
- 2 whole eggs
- 3 egg whites
- Red, green, blue and yellow food coloring

Directions:

1. Mix the butter and sugar in a container until fluffy and creamy.
2. Stir in the eggs, egg whites, vanilla and sour cream and stir thoroughly for a few minutes.
3. Mix the flour with baking powder, baking soda and salt then fold it in the batter.
4. Divide the batter into 4 smaller containers then add a drop of food colouring into each container and stir gently using a spoon in each batch of batter.
5. Spoon the colourful batter into a 9-inch cake pan coated with baking paper.
6. Use a toothpick to swirl the batter around until colours are blended.
7. Pre-heat the oven and bake at 350F for around forty minutes.
8. Let the cake cool in the pan then serve, sliced.

Nutritional Content of One Serving:

Calories: 433 | Fat: 22.0g | Protein: 6.0g | Carbohydrates: 54.8g

Raspberry Chocolate Cake

Total Time Taken: 1 ¼ hours

Yield: 10 Servings

Ingredients:

- ½ cup butter, melted
- ½ teaspoon baking powder
- ½ teaspoon salt
- 1 ¼ cups all-purpose flour
- 1 cup white sugar
- 1 teaspoon vanilla extract
- 2 cups fresh raspberries
- 3 oz. dark chocolate, melted
- 6 eggs

Directions:

1. Mix the eggs and sugar in a container until its volume increases to almost three times it was.
2. Stir in the melted butter and chocolate, as well as vanilla.
3. Fold in the baking powder and salt then put in the raspberries and stir lightly.
4. Pour the batter in a 9-inch round cake pan and preheat your oven and bake at 350F for around forty minutes or until a toothpick inserted into the center of the cake comes out clean.
5. Let cool in the pan then serve, sliced.

Nutritional Content of One Serving:

Calories: 311 | Fat: 14.7g | Protein: 6.0g | Carbohydrates: 40.3g

Raspberry Chocolate Mud Cake

Total Time Taken: 1 ½ hours

Yield: 12 Servings

Ingredients:

- ½ cup buttermilk
- ½ cup cocoa powder
- ½ cup heavy cream
- ½ teaspoon salt
- 1 ½ cups fresh raspberries
- 1 ½ cups white sugar
- 1 cup butter, softened
- 1 cup dark chocolate chips
- 1 cup hot water
- 2 cups all-purpose flour
- 2 tablespoons brandy
- 2 teaspoons baking powder
- 3 eggs

Directions:

1. Mix the butter and chocolate chips in a heatproof container and place over a hot water bath. Melt them together until the desired smoothness is achieved.
2. Stir in the sugar and hot water and mix thoroughly.

3. Put in the buttermilk, cream, eggs and brandy.
4. Fold in the dry ingredients and mix thoroughly.
5. Put in the raspberries and pour the batter in a 9-inch round cake pan coated with baking paper.
6. Pre-heat the oven and bake at 350F for 50 minutes.
7. Let the cake cool in the pan and serve, sliced.

Nutritional Content of One Serving:
Calories: 415 | Fat: 21.8g | Protein: 5.6g | Carbohydrates: 52.5g

Raspberry Ganache Cake

Total Time Taken: 1 ¼ hours
Yield: 8 Servings
Ingredients:
Cake:

- ¼ teaspoon salt
- ½ cup butter, softened
- ½ cup white sugar
- 1 cup all-purpose flour
- 1 cup fresh raspberries
- 1 teaspoon baking powder
- 4 eggs

Ganache:

- ½ cup heavy cream
- 1 cup dark chocolate chips

Directions:
1. For the cake, combine the butter and sugar in a container until fluffy. Put in the eggs, one at a time, then mix in the flour, salt and baking powder.
2. Spoon the batter in a 8-inch round cake pan coated with baking paper.
3. Top with raspberries and preheat your oven and bake at 350F for around forty minutes or until it rises significantly and starts to appear golden-brown.
4. Let the cake cool in the pan then move to a platter.
5. For the ganache, bring the cream to the boiling point in a saucepan. Turn off the heat and mix in the chocolate. Combine until melted.
6. Sprinkle the ganache over the cake and serve the cake chilled.

Nutritional Content of One Serving:
Calories: 341 | Fat: 20.7g | Protein: 5.8g | Carbohydrates: 37.0g

Raspberry Lemon Olive Oil Cake

Total Time Taken: 1 hour
Yield: 10 Servings
Ingredients:

- ¼ cup butter, softened
- ¼ cup whole milk
- ¼ teaspoon baking soda
- ½ teaspoon salt
- ¾ cup extra virgin olive oil
- 1 ¾ cups all-purpose flour
- 1 cup fresh raspberries
- 1 cup white sugar
- 1 teaspoon baking powder
- 2 tablespoons lemon zest
- 4 eggs

Directions:
1. Mix the flour, baking powder, baking soda and salt in a container or platter.
2. In a separate container, mix the oil, butter and sugar and mix thoroughly. Stir in the eggs, one at a time, then put in the milk and lemon zest.
3. Fold in the dry ingredients then put in the raspberries.
4. Spoon the batter in a round cake pan coated with baking paper and preheat your oven and bake at 350F for around forty minutes or until a toothpick inserted into the center of the cake comes out clean. The cake tastes best chilled.

Nutritional Content of One Serving:
Calories: 361 | Fat: 22.0g | Protein: 4.9g | Carbohydrates: 39.1g

Raspberry Matcha Cake

Total Time Taken: 1 ¼ hours
Yield: 10 Servings
Ingredients:

- ½ teaspoon salt
- 1 ½ cups all-purpose flour
- 1 cup fresh raspberries
- 1 tablespoons matcha powder
- 1 teaspoon vanilla extract
- 2 teaspoons baking powder
- 2/3 cup butter, softened
- 2/3 cup white sugar
- 4 eggs

Directions:
1. Sift the flour, matcha powder, baking powder and salt in a container.
2. Mix the butter and sugar until fluffy and creamy.
3. Put in the eggs, one at a time, and mix thoroughly after each addition. Stir in the vanilla then fold in the flour.
4. Put in the raspberries then spoon the batter in a loaf cake pan coated with baking paper.
5. Pre-heat the oven and bake at 350F for around forty minutes or until a toothpick inserted into the center of the cake comes out clean.
6. *The cake tastes best chilled.*

Nutritional Content of One Serving:
Calories: 262 | Fat: 14.3g | Protein: 4.4g | Carbohydrates: 30.3g

Raspberry Ricotta Cake

Total Time Taken: 1 hour
Yield: 10 Servings
Ingredients:

- ¼ cup cocoa powder
- ¼ teaspoon salt
- ½ cup butter, softened
- ¾ cup white sugar
- 1 cup hot water
- 1 cup raspberries
- 1 cup ricotta cheese
- 2 cups all-purpose flour
- 2 teaspoons baking powder

Directions:

1. Mix the ricotta cheese, butter and sugar in a container until creamy.
2. Put in the water and mix thoroughly.
3. Fold in the flour, cocoa powder, baking powder and salt.
4. Put in the raspberries then spoon the batter in a 9-inch round cake pan coated with baking paper.
5. Pre-heat the oven and bake at 350F for forty minutes or until a toothpick inserted into the center of the cake comes out clean.
6. The cake tastes best chilled.

Nutritional Content of One Serving:
Calories: 275 | Fat: 11.8g | Protein: 6.0g | Carbohydrates: 38.5g

Rhubarb Upside Down Cake

Total Time Taken: 1 ¼ hours
Yield: 10 Servings
Ingredients:

- ½ cup sour cream
- ½ cup white sugar
- ½ teaspoon salt
- ¾ cup butter, softened
- ¾ cup white sugar
- 1 ½ teaspoons baking powder
- 1 teaspoon vanilla extract
- 2 cups all-purpose flour
- 3 eggs
- 4 rhubarb stalks, peeled and sliced

Directions:

1. Position the stalks of rhubarb in a 9-inch round cake pan coated with baking paper.
2. Top with ½ cup white sugar.
3. Mix the butter with
4. 1 cup sugar until fluffy and pale.
5. Put in the eggs and sour cream and mix thoroughly.
6. Stir in the vanilla then fold in the flour, baking powder and salt.
7. Pour the batter in the pan and preheat your oven and bake at 350F for about forty minutes.
8. When finished, flip the cake upside down on a platter.

Nutritional Content of One Serving:
Calories: 357 | Fat: 17.8g | Protein: 4.9g | Carbohydrates: 46.0g

Rich Vanilla Cake

Total Time Taken: 1 hour
Yield: 10 Servings
Ingredients:

- ½ teaspoon salt
- 1 cup butter, softened
- 1 cup white sugar
- 1 tablespoon vanilla extract
- 2 cups all-purpose flour
- 2 egg whites
- 2 teaspoons baking powder
- 6 egg yolks

Directions:

1. Mix the butter, sugar and vanilla in a container until fluffy and creamy.
2. Put in the egg yolks and whole eggs, one at a time, stirring thoroughly after each addition.
3. Fold in the flour, baking powder and salt then spoon the batter in a 9-inch round cake pan coated with baking paper.
4. Pre-heat the oven and bake at 350F for around forty minutes or until a toothpick inserted into the center of the cake comes out clean.
5. Let the cake cool in the pan before you serve.

Nutritional Content of One Serving:
Calories: 369 | Fat: 21.4g | Protein: 5.1g | Carbohydrates: 40.1g

Rum Pineapple Upside Down Cake

Total Time Taken: 1 ¼ hours
Yield: 10 Servings
Ingredients:

- ¼ cup butter, melted
- ¼ cup light rum
- ¼ teaspoon salt
- 1 ½ teaspoons baking powder
- 1 can pineapple rings, drained
- 1 cup white sugar
- 2 cups all-purpose flour
- 4 eggs

Directions:

1. Position the pineapple rings at the bottom of a 9-inch round cake pan coated with baking paper.
2. Mix the eggs and sugar in a container until volume increases to twice what it was.
3. Stir in the rum and melted butter then fold in the flour, baking powder and salt.

4. Pour the batter over the pineapple and preheat your oven and bake at 350F for around forty minutes.
5. When finished, flip it over on a platter and let cool before you serve.

Nutritional Content of One Serving:
Calories: 254 | Fat: 6.6g | Protein: 4.9g | Carbohydrates: 41.7g

Snickerdoodle Bundt Cake

Total Time Taken: 1 ½ hours
Yield: 12 Servings
Ingredients:
Filling:

- 1 cup white sugar
- 1 tablespoon cinnamon powder

Cake:

- ½ teaspoon baking soda
- ½ teaspoon salt
- 1 cup butter, softened
- 1 cup sour cream
- 1 cup white sugar
- 1 teaspoon baking powder
- 1 teaspoon ground ginger
- 2 ½ cups all-purpose flour
- 2 tablespoons dark brown sugar
- 3 eggs

Directions:
1. For the filling, combine the sugar with cinnamon in a container.
2. For the cake, sift the flour, ginger, baking powder, baking soda and salt.
3. Mix the butter and sugars in a container until fluffy and light.
4. Put in the eggs, one at a time, then mix in the sour cream.
5. Fold in the flour then spoon half of the batter in a greased Bundt cake pan. Drizzle with the cinnamon sugar mixture then top with the rest of the batter.
6. Pre-heat the oven and bake at 350F for about forty-five minutes or until a golden-brown colour is achieved and a toothpick inserted into the center of the cake comes out clean.
7. *The cake tastes best chilled.*

Nutritional Content of One Serving:
Calories: 419 | Fat: 20.7g | Protein: 4.9g | Carbohydrates: 55.9g

Sour Cherry Chocolate Cake

Total Time Taken: 1 ¼ hours
Yield: 10 Servings
Ingredients:

- ¼ cup whole milk
- ½ cup cocoa powder
- ½ teaspoon salt
- 1 cup all-purpose flour
- 1 cup butter, softened
- 1 cup heavy cream, whipped
- 1 cup sour cherries, pitted
- 1 cup white sugar
- 1 teaspoon baking powder
- 1 teaspoon vanilla extract
- 4 eggs

Directions:
1. Sift the flour with cocoa, salt and baking powder.
2. Mix the butter with sugar and vanilla until creamy. Put in the eggs, one at a time, then fold in the flour mixture.
3. Put in the cherries then spoon the batter in a 9-inch round cake pan coated with baking paper.
4. Pre-heat the oven and bake at 350F for around forty minutes or until a toothpick comes out clean after being inserted into the center of the cake.
5. Let the cake cool then move to a platter and cover it in whipped cream.
6. Serve fresh or place in your refrigerator.

Nutritional Content of One Serving:
Calories: 373 | Fat: 25.5g | Protein: 5.0g | Carbohydrates: 35.0g

Spiced Pumpkin Sheet Cake

Total Time Taken: 1 ¼ hours
Yield: 16 Servings
Ingredients:

- ¼ teaspoon baking soda
- ½ cup walnuts, chopped
- ½ teaspoon ground cloves
- ½ teaspoon ground star anise
- ½ teaspoon salt
- 1 ½ cups pumpkin puree
- 1 ½ cups white sugar
- 1 cup canola oil
- 1 teaspoon cinnamon powder
- 1 teaspoon ground ginger
- 2 cups all-purpose flour
- 2 teaspoons baking powder
- 4 eggs

Directions:
1. Sift the flour, baking powder, baking soda, salt and spices in a container.
2. Mix the sugar, canola oil and eggs in a container until pale and fluffy.
3. Stir in the pumpkin puree then incorporate the flour, ½ cup at a time, mixing gently using a spatula.
4. Fold in the walnuts then spoon the batter in a 10x10 inch rectangle pan coated with baking paper.
5. Pre-heat the oven and bake at 350F for around forty minutes or until a toothpick inserted into the center of the cake comes out clean.

6. The cake tastes best chilled, cut into small squares.

Nutritional Content of One Serving:
Calories: 297 | Fat: 17.3g | Protein: 4.2g | Carbohydrates: 33.5g

Spiced Walnut Cake

Total Time Taken: 1 hour
Yield: 8 Servings
Ingredients:
3 eggs

- ¼ cup canola oil
- ½ teaspoon ground cardamom
- ½ teaspoon ground ginger
- ½ teaspoon salt
- ¾ cup all-purpose flour
- 1 cup ground walnuts
- 1 cup white sugar
- 1 teaspoon baking soda
- 1 teaspoon cinnamon powder

Directions:

1. Mix the eggs and sugar in a container until fluffy and volume increases to twice what it was.
2. Stir in the canola oil then fold in the walnuts, cinnamon, ginger, cardamom, flour, salt and baking soda.
3. Pour the batter in a 8-inch round cake pan coated with baking paper.
4. Pre-heat the oven and bake at 350F for around forty minutes or until it rises completely and is aromatic.
5. Let the cake cool in the pan and serve, sliced.

Nutritional Content of One Serving:
Calories: 318 | Fat: 17.8g | Protein: 7.1g | Carbohydrates: 35.8g

Spicy Chocolate Cake

Total Time Taken: 1 hour
Yield: Servings 6
Ingredients:

- ¼ cup canola oil
- ¼ teaspoon cinnamon powder
- ½ cup cocoa powder
- ½ teaspoon salt
- 1 ½ cups all-purpose flour
- 1 cup hot coffee
- 1 teaspoon baking soda
- 1 teaspoon vanilla extract
- 1/2 teaspoon chili powder
- 2 oz. dark chocolate, chopped

Directions:

1. Sift the flour with cocoa powder, chili, cinnamon, baking soda and salt.
2. Mix the canola oil with coffee and chocolate and stir until it melts completely.
3. Put in the vanilla, then fold in the flour mixture.
4. Pour the batter in a 9-inch round cake pan covered with parchment paper and preheat your oven and bake at 350F for around forty minutes or until a toothpick comes out clean after being inserted into the center of the cake.
5. The cake tastes best chilled.

Nutritional Content of One Serving:
Calories: 264 | Fat: 13.2g | Protein: 5.3g | Carbohydrates: 33.6g

Strawberry Cake

Total Time Taken: 1 ½ hours
Yield: 12 Servings
Ingredients:
Cake:

- ½ cup canola oil
- ½ cup coconut milk
- ½ teaspoon salt
- 1 cup white sugar
- 1 teaspoon vanilla extract
- 2 cups all-purpose flour
- 2 teaspoons baking powder
- 4 eggs

Strawberry buttercream:

- ¼ cup strawberry puree
- 1 cup butter
- 3 cups powdered sugar

Directions:

1. For the cake, combine the flour, baking powder and salt in a container.
2. In a separate container, combine the sugar, canola oil and eggs in a container until volume increases to twice what it was.
3. Stir in the milk and vanilla then fold in the dry ingredients.
4. Spoon the batter in two 9-inch circular cake pans and preheat your oven and bake at 350F for half an hour.
5. Let the cakes cool in the pan then level them up.
6. For the buttercream, combine the butter and sugar in a container until firm and fluffy.
7. Stir in the strawberry puree and mix thoroughly.
8. Fill the cake with half of the buttercream then use the rest of the buttercream to cover the cake.
9. Serve immediately or place in your refrigerator.

Nutritional Content of One Serving:
Calories: 522 | Fat: 28.6g | Protein: 4.4g | Carbohydrates: 64.6g

Strawberry Crumble Cake

Total Time Taken: 1 ¼ hours

Yield: 12 Servings
Ingredients:
Cake:

- ¼ cup canola oil
- ¼ teaspoon salt
- ½ teaspoon baking powder
- 1 ½ cups all-purpose flour
- 1 cup plain yogurt
- 1 cup white sugar
- 1 teaspoon vanilla extract
- 2 cups fresh strawberries, sliced
- 6 eggs

Crumble:

- ¼ cup chilled butter
- ½ cup all-purpose flour
- 2 tablespoons white sugar

Directions:

1. For the cake, combine the eggs, sugar and vanilla in a container until fluffy and twofold in volume at least.
2. Stir in the yogurt and oil then fold in the flour, baking powder and salt.
3. Pour the batter in a 9-inch round cake pan coated with baking paper.
4. Top with strawberries.
5. For the streusel, combine all the ingredients in a container until grainy.
6. Top the cake with streusel and preheat your oven and bake at 350F for 45 minutes or until a toothpick comes out clean after being inserted into the center of the cake.
7. *The cake tastes best chilled.*

Nutritional Content of One Serving:
Calories: 275 | Fat: 11.1g | Protein: 6.3g | Carbohydrates: 38.2g

Strawberry Lemon Olive Oil Cake

Total Time Taken: 1 ¼ hours
Yield: 10 Servings
Ingredients:

- ¼ teaspoon salt
- ¾ cup olive oil
- ¾ cup white sugar
- 1 ¼ cups all-purpose flour
- 1 ½ cups strawberries, sliced
- 1 lemon, zested and juiced
- 1 teaspoon baking powder
- 4 eggs

Directions:

1. Mix the eggs, oil and sugar in a container until fluffy and pale.
2. Put in the lemon zest and juice and mix thoroughly.
3. Fold in the flour, baking powder and salt then spoon the batter in a 9-inch round cake pan coated with baking paper.
4. Top with strawberries and preheat your oven and bake at 350F for about forty minutes.
5. Let the cake cool in the pan before you serve.

Nutritional Content of One Serving:
Calories: 277 | Fat: 17.1g | Protein: 4.0g | Carbohydrates: 29.5g

Strawberry Polenta Cake

Total Time Taken: 1 ¼ hours
Yield: 10 Servings
Ingredients:

- ¼ cup butter, melted
- ¼ teaspoon salt
- ½ cup white sugar
- 1 cup polenta flour
- 1 teaspoon baking soda
- 1 teaspoon vanilla extract
- 2 cups strawberries, sliced
- 2 cups water
- 2 cups whole milk
- 2 tablespoons all-purpose flour

Directions:

1. Mix the polenta flour, flour, salt and baking soda in a container.
2. Stir in the milk, water, sugar, vanilla and melted butter.
3. Pour the batter in a 8x8-inch and top with strawberry slices.
4. Pre-heat the oven and bake at 350F for around forty minutes or until a toothpick inserted into the center of the cake comes out clean.
5. When finished, take it out of the oven, let cool down then cut into small squares.
6. *Serve immediately.*

Nutritional Content of One Serving:
Calories: 147 | Fat: 6.4g | Protein: 2.4g | Carbohydrates: 20.7g

Strawberry Yogurt Cake

Total Time Taken: 1 hour
Yield: 8 Servings
Ingredients:

- ½ cup butter, softened
- 1 cup all-purpose flour
- 1 cup strawberries, sliced
- 1 cup white sugar
- 1 teaspoon baking powder
- 1 teaspoon vanilla extract
- 1/2 cup plain yogurt
- 3 eggs

Directions:

1. Mix the butter and sugar until softened and creamy.
2. Put in the eggs, one at a time, then mix in the yogurt and vanilla.

3. Fold in the flour and baking powder using a spatula then put in the strawberries.
4. Pour the batter in a round cake pan coated with baking paper.
5. Pre-heat the oven and bake at 350F for about forty minutes or until a toothpick inserted into the center of the cake comes out clean.
6. Let the cake cool in the pan before you serve.

Nutritional Content of One Serving:
Calories: 295 | Fat: 13.5g | Protein: 4.8g | Carbohydrates: 39.9g

Sultana Cake

Total Time Taken: 1 ½ hours
Yield: 10 Servings
Ingredients:

- ¼ cup orange marmalade
- ¼ teaspoon salt
- ½ cup brandy
- ½ cup butter, softened
- 1 ½ cups sultanas
- 1 cup all-purpose flour
- 1 cup white sugar
- 1 teaspoon baking soda
- 2 eggs
- 2 tablespoons dark brown sugar

Directions:

1. Mix the sultanas with the brandy and allow to soak up for about half an hour.
2. Mix the butter, sugars and marmalade in a container until creamy.
3. Put in the eggs and mix thoroughly.
4. Fold in the flour, salt and baking soda then put in the sultanas.
5. Spoon the batter in a 8-inch round cake pan coated with baking paper.
6. Pre-heat the oven and bake at 350F for about fifty minutes or until a toothpick inserted into the center of the cake comes out clean.
7. Let the cake cool down before you serve.

Nutritional Content of One Serving:
Calories: 262 | Fat: 10.2g | Protein: 2.7g | Carbohydrates: 40.7g

Summer Fruit Cake

Total Time Taken: 1 ¼ hours
Yield: 12 Servings
Ingredients:

- ½ cup butter, softened
- ½ cup canola oil
- 1 cup all-purpose flour
- 1 cup cherries, pitted
- 1 cup ground almonds
- 1 cup mixed berries
- 1 cup white sugar
- 1 teaspoon baking powder
- 1 teaspoon vanilla extract
- 6 eggs

Directions:

1. Mix the butter, oil and sugar in a container until creamy and fluffy. Put in the vanilla and eggs, one at a time, and mix thoroughly.
2. Stir in the almonds, flour and baking powder then pour the batter in a 9-inch round cake pan coated with baking paper.
3. Top with berries and cherries and preheat your oven and bake at 350F for 40- 45 minutes or until it rises significantly and starts to appear golden-brown.
4. Let the cake cool in the pan and serve, sliced.

Nutritional Content of One Serving:
Calories: 341 | Fat: 23.0g | Protein: 5.7g | Carbohydrates: 29.9g

Sweet Potato Bundt Cake

Total Time Taken: 1 hour
Yield: 10 Servings
Ingredients:

- 1 cup sweet potato puree
- 2 eggs
- ½ cup sour cream
- ¼ cup canola oil
- 1 teaspoon vanilla extract
- 2 cups all-purpose flour
- 2 teaspoons baking powder
- ½ teaspoon salt
- ½ cup dark chocolate chips
- 3/4 cup maple syrup

Directions:

1. Mix the potato puree, maple syrup, eggs, sour cream, canola oil and vanilla in a container.
2. Stir in the remaining ingredients then spoon the batter in a greased Bundt cake pan.
3. Pre-heat the oven and bake at 350F for about forty minutes or until a toothpick comes out clean after being inserted into the center of the cake.
4. Let the cake cool in the pan then serve, sliced.

Nutritional Content of One Serving:
Calories: 294 | Fat: 10.7g | Protein: 5.0g | Carbohydrates: 45.9g

Tahini Cake

Total Time Taken: 1 ¼ hours
Yield: 10 Servings
Ingredients:

- ½ cup butter, softened
- ½ cup tahini paste
- ½ teaspoon baking soda
- ½ teaspoon salt

- 1 cup buttermilk
- 1 cup white sugar
- 1 teaspoon baking powder
- 1 teaspoon vanilla extract
- 2 cups all-purpose flour
- 2 eggs

Directions:

1. **Mix** the tahini paste, butter and sugar in a container and give it a good mix.
2. **Stir in** the eggs, one at a time, then put in the vanilla and buttermilk.
3. Fold in the flour, baking powder, baking soda and salt then spoon the batter in a round cake pan coated with baking paper.
4. Pre-heat the oven and bake at 350F **for about forty minutes** or until the cake is well risen and seems golden brown.
5. Let the cake cool in the pan and serve, sliced.

Nutritional Content of One Serving:

Calories: 343 | Fat: 17.0g | Protein: 6.6g | Carbohydrates: 43.1g

The Ultimate Chocolate Cake

Total Time Taken: 1 ¼ hours

Yield: 14 Servings

Ingredients:

Cake:

- ¼ cup canola oil
- ½ cup cocoa powder
- ½ teaspoon salt
- 1 ½ cups white sugar
- 1 cup butter, softened
- 1 cup buttermilk
- 2 ½ cups all-purpose flour
- 2 egg yolks
- 2 teaspoons baking powder
- 4 eggs

Frosting:

- 1 ½ cups dark chocolate chips
- 1 cup heavy cream

Directions:

1. Mix the butter and sugar in a container until creamy and fluffy.
2. Stir in the eggs and egg yolks and mix thoroughly.
3. Put in the buttermilk and oil and mix thoroughly then fold in the dry ingredients.
4. Pour the batter in a 10-inch round cake pan and preheat your oven and bake at 350F for 45 minutes or until the toothpick inserted in the center of the cake comes out clean.
5. Let the cake cool in the pan then move to a platter.
6. For the frosting, bring the cream to the boiling point then turn off the heat and put in the chocolate. let the frosting cool in your refrigerator for a few hours then whip it using an electric mixer until fluffy.
7. Sprinkle the chocolate frosting over the cake and serve it fresh.

Nutritional Content of One Serving:

Calories: 442 | Fat: 26.3g | Protein: 6.6g | Carbohydrates: 50.3g

Tiramisu Cake

Total Time Taken: 2 hours

Yield: 12 Servings

Ingredients:

- ¼ cup Grand Marnier
- 1 cup powdered sugar
- 1 tablespoon vanilla extract
- 10 oz. ladyfingers
- 2 cups brewed coffee
- 2 cups heavy cream, whipped
- 2 cups mascarpone cheese

Directions:

1. Coat a 9-inch round cake pan using plastic wrap.
2. Mix the mascarpone cheese with sugar then fold in the whipped cream.
3. Mix the coffee and Grand Marnier in a container.
4. Immerse the ladyfingers in the coffee mixture and layer them at the bottom of the pan.
5. Top with 1/3 of the cream, followed by an additional layer of ladyfingers.
6. Carry on until you run out of ingredients and place in your fridge at least an hour.
7. *The cake tastes best chilled.*

Nutritional Content of One Serving:

Calories: 285 | Fat: 14.9g | Protein: 7.6g | Carbohydrates: 26.0g

Tropical Carrot Cake

Total Time Taken: 1 ½ hours

Yield: 16 Servings

Ingredients:

Cake:

- ¼ cup dark brown sugar
- 1 cup vegetable oil
- ½ cup chopped walnuts
- 1 cup shredded coconut **Frosting:**
- ½ teaspoon ground cloves
- 1 cup white sugar
- ½ teaspoon ground ginger
- ½ teaspoon salt
- 1 cup butter, softened
- 1 cup cream cheese, softened
- 2 ½ cups powdered sugar
- 1 cup crushed pineapple (with juice)
- 1 teaspoon baking powder
- 1 teaspoon cinnamon powder

- 1 teaspoon vanilla extract
- 1 teaspoon vanilla extract
- 4 carrots, grated
- 2 cups all-purpose flour
- 1 teaspoon baking soda
- 4 eggs

Directions:

1. For the cake, combine the flour, baking soda, baking powder, spices and salt in a container.
2. Combine the sugars, oil, eggs and vanilla in a container and stir thoroughly until volume increases to twice what it was.
3. Stir in the carrots, pineapple, walnuts and coconut then put in the dry ingredients.
4. Pour the batter in two 9-inch cake pans and preheat your oven and bake at 350F for around forty minutes or until it rises and looks golden brown.
5. Let the cakes cool in the pans then level them and set aside for later.
6. For the frosting, combine the cream cheese, butter, sugar and vanilla in a container for minimum five minutes until firm and fluffy.
7. Use half of the frosting to fill the cakes and the second half to garnish them.

Nutritional Content of One Serving:
Calories: 529 | Fat: 35.5g | Protein: 5.5g | Carbohydrates: 50.1g

Vanilla Cardamom Cake

Total Time Taken: 1 ¼ hours
Yield: 12 Servings
Ingredients:
Cake:

- ¼ teaspoon salt
- ½ cup canola oil
- 1 ½ cups all-purpose flour
- 1 cup white sugar
- 1 teaspoon baking powder
- 1 teaspoon cardamom powder
- 6 eggs

Frosting:

- ½ cup butter, softened
- 1 ½ cups powdered sugar
- 1 cup cream cheese
- 1 teaspoon vanilla extract

Directions:

1. For the cake, sift the flour with baking powder, salt and cardamom.
2. Mix the eggs with sugar until fluffy and pale.
3. Put in the oil and mix thoroughly then fold in the flour.
4. Pour the batter in a 9-inch round cake pan coated with baking paper.
5. Pre-heat the oven and bake at 350F for about forty minutes.
6. When finished, allow the cake to cool in the pan then cut it in half along the length.
7. For the frosting, combine the butter and cream cheese in a container until fluffy. Put in the vanilla and sugar and continue mixing for minimum five minutes until pale.
8. Use half of the frosting as filling and the second half to cover the cake.
9. *Serve the cake fresh.*

Nutritional Content of One Serving:
Calories: 427 | Fat: 25.9g | Protein: 5.9g | Carbohydrates: 44.6g

Vanilla Funfetti Cake

Total Time Taken: 1 ½ hours
Yield: 12 Servings
Ingredients:
Cake:

- ½ cup sprinkles
- ½ teaspoon salt
- 1 ½ teaspoons baking powder
- 1 cup butter, softened
- 1 cup sour cream
- 1 cup white sugar
- 1 teaspoon vanilla extract
- 2 cups all-purpose flour
- 3 eggs

Frosting:

- ½ cup butter, softened
- 1 ½ cups powdered sugar
- 1 teaspoon vanilla extract

Directions:

1. For the cake, combine the butter and sugar in a container until fluffy and creamy.
2. Put in the eggs and vanilla and stir thoroughly for a few minutes.
3. Stir in the sour cream then fold in the flour, baking powder and salt, as well as sprinkles.
4. Spoon the batter in a 9-inch round cake pan coated with baking paper.
5. Pre-heat the oven and bake at 350F for about forty minutes or until it rises significantly and starts to appear golden-brown.
6. For the frosting, combine the butter, sugar and vanilla and stir thoroughly until fluffy and
7. pale.
8. Top the cake with frosting and serve it fresh.

Nutritional Content of One Serving:
Calories: 464 | Fat: 28.3g | Protein: 4.4g | Carbohydrates: 50.0g

Vanilla Genoise Cake

Total Time Taken: 1 hour
Yield: 8 Servings
Ingredients:
6 eggs

- ¼ teaspoon baking powder
- ¼ teaspoon salt
- ¾ cup white sugar
- 1 cup all-purpose flour
- 1 teaspoon vanilla extract

Directions:

1. Mix the eggs, sugar and vanilla in a container until fluffy and light.
2. Fold in the flour, salt and baking powder then spoon the batter in a 8-inch round cake pan coated with baking paper.
3. Pre-heat the oven and bake at 350F for about half an hour or until it rises significantly and starts to appear golden-brown.
4. Let the cake cool down before you serve.

Nutritional Content of One Serving:

Calories: 176 | Fat: 3.4g | Protein: 5.8g | Carbohydrates: 31.1g

Vanilla Strawberry Cake

Total Time Taken: 1 ½ hours

Yield: 10 Servings

Ingredients:

Cake:

- ¼ cup sour cream
- ½ cup butter, softened
- ½ cup whole milk
- ½ teaspoon baking soda
- ½ teaspoon salt
- 1 ½ cups all-purpose flour
- 1 cup white sugar
- 1 teaspoon baking powder
- 1 teaspoon vanilla extract
- 4 egg whites

Filling:

- ½ cup butter, softened
- 1 cup fresh strawberries, sliced
- 2 cups powdered sugar
- 2 teaspoons vanilla extract

Directions:

1. For the cake, sift the flour with baking powder, baking soda and salt in a container.
2. Put in the sugar and butter and stir until grainy.
3. Combine the egg whites, milk and sour cream, as well as vanilla in a container. Pour this mixture over the dry ingredients and stir only until blended.
4. Spoon the batter in two 8-inch circular cake pans coated with baking paper.
5. For the filling, combine the butter with sugar for five minutes until fluffy and creamy. Put in the vanilla and mix thoroughly.
6. Fill the cake with the buttercream and strawberry slices.
7. Serve it fresh.

Nutritional Content of One Serving:

Calories: 435 | Fat: 20.3g | Protein: 4.2g | Carbohydrates: 60.6g

Vanilla White Chocolate Chip Cake

Total Time Taken: 1 ¼ hours

Yield: 12 Servings

Ingredients:

- ½ teaspoon salt
- 1 ½ teaspoons baking powder
- 1 cup butter, softened
- 1 cup white chocolate chips
- 1 cup white sugar
- 1 cup whole milk
- 1 tablespoon vanilla extract
- 2 cups all-purpose flour
- 4 eggs

Directions:

1. Mix the butter and sugar in a container until fluffy and pale.
2. Stir in the eggs, one at a time, then put in the vanilla and milk.
3. Stir in the flour, baking powder and salt then fold in the chocolate chips.
4. Spoon the batter in a 9-inch round cake pan coated with baking paper.
5. Pre-heat the oven and bake at 350F for about forty minutes.
6. Let the cake cool in the pan and serve, sliced.

Nutritional Content of One Serving:

Calories: 387 | Fat: 22.2g | Protein: 5.6g | Carbohydrates: 42.4g

Victoria Sponge Cake With Strawberries

Total Time Taken: 1 ¼ hours

Yield: 8 Servings

Ingredients:

- ¼ teaspoon salt
- 1 ¼ cups all-purpose flour
- 1 cup butter, softened
- 1 cup fresh strawberries, sliced
- 1 cup heavy cream, whipped
- 1 cup white sugar
- 1 teaspoon baking powder
- 4 eggs

Directions:

1. Mix the butter and sugar in a container until light and creamy.
2. Stir in the eggs, one at a time, then fold in the flour, salt and baking powder.
3. Spoon the batter in a 9-inch round cake pan covered with parchment paper and preheat your oven and bake at 350F for about half an hour or until it rises significantly and starts to appear golden-brown.

4. Let the cake cool down then take it out of the pan and cut it in half along the length.
5. Fill the cake with whipped cream and strawberries and garnish it with a dust of powdered sugar.

Nutritional Content of One Serving:
Calories: 458 | Fat: 31.0g | Protein: 5.5g | Carbohydrates: 42.2g

Walnut Banana Cake

Total Time Taken: 1 ¼ hours
Yield: 10 Servings
Ingredients:

- ¼ cup whole milk
- ½ teaspoon salt
- 1 cup butter, softened
- 1 cup ground walnuts
- 1 cup light brown sugar
- 1 teaspoon cinnamon powder
- 2 cups all-purpose flour
- 2 teaspoons baking soda
- 3 ripe bananas, mashed
- 4 eggs

Directions:

1. Mix the flour, walnuts, baking soda, salt and cinnamon in a container.
2. In a separate container, combine the butter and sugar until creamy, then put in the eggs, one at a time.
3. Put in the milk and bananas then fold in the flour mixture.
4. Spoon the batter into a 10-inch round cake pan coated with baking paper.
5. Pre-heat the oven and bake at 350F or until a toothpick inserted into the center of the cake comes out clean.
6. Let the cake cool completely and serve, sliced.

Nutritional Content of One Serving:
Calories: 446 | Fat: 28.1g | Protein: 8.6g | Carbohydrates: 43.1g

Walnut Carrot Cake

Total Time Taken: 1 ½ hours
Yield: 16 Servings
Ingredients:
Cake:

- ½ cup ground walnuts
- ½ teaspoon salt
- 1 cup canola oil
- 1 cup chopped walnuts
- 1 cup crushed pineapple
- 1 cup white sugar
- 1 teaspoon all-spice powder
- 1 teaspoon baking powder
- 1 teaspoon baking soda
- 1 teaspoon cinnamon powder
- 2 cups all-purpose flour
- 2 cups grated carrots
- 3 eggs

Frosting:

- ¼ cup butter
- 1 cup cream cheese, softened
- 3 cups powdered sugar

Directions:

1. To prepare the cake, combine the dry ingredients in a container and the wet ingredients in another container.
2. Pour the wet ingredients over the dry ones and mix using a spatula.
3. Pour the batter in 9-inch round cake pan coated with baking paper.
4. Preheat your oven and bake the cake at 350F for about forty minutes or until they pass the toothpick test.
5. Let the cakes cool completely.
6. For the frosting, combine the cream cheese and butter in a container until creamy.
7. Put in the sugar, progressively, stirring thoroughly after each addition.
8. Whip the frosting thoroughly until fluffy.
9. Fill the cake with 1/3 of the frosting and cover it with the rest of the cream cheese frosting.
10. Serve the cake fresh or place in your refrigerator.

Nutritional Content of One Serving:
Calories: 483 | Fat: 29.5g | Protein: 6.8g | Carbohydrates: 51.3g

Walnut Coffee Cake

Total Time Taken: 2 hours
Yield: 16 Servings
Ingredients:
Walnut cake:

- ¼ cup whole milk
- ½ teaspoon salt
- 1 cup butter, softened
- 1 cup ground walnuts
- 1 cup white sugar
- 1 teaspoon vanilla extract
- 2 cups all-purpose flour
- 2 teaspoons baking powder
- 4 eggs

Coffee buttercream:

- 1 cup butter, softened
- 1 teaspoon vanilla extract
- 2 ½ cups powdered sugar
- 2 teaspoons instant coffee

Directions:

1. For the cake, combine the flour, baking powder, walnuts and salt in a container.

2. In a separate container, combine the butter and sugar until creamy. Stir in the eggs, one at a time, then put in the milk and vanilla.
3. Fold in the flour and stir lightly using a spatula.
4. Pour the batter in a round cake pan coated with baking paper and preheat your oven and bake at 350F for around forty minutes.
5. Let the cake cool in the pan then move to a platter.
6. For the buttercream, combine the butter until creamy and light. Put in the sugar, progressively and stir thoroughly for a few minutes until firm.
7. Mix the vanilla with the coffee then add it into the buttercream. Stir thoroughly to mix.
8. Cover the cake with the buttercream and serve it fresh.

Nutritional Content of One Serving:
Calories: 449 | Fat: 29.0g | Protein: 5.2g | Carbohydrates: 44.5g

Walnut Honey Pound Cake

Total Time Taken: 1 ¼ hours
Yield: 12 Servings
Ingredients:

- ½ cup butter, softened
- ½ teaspoon salt
- 1 ½ cups walnuts, chopped
- 1 cup honey
- 1 cup whole milk
- 1 teaspoon vanilla extract
- 2 cups all-purpose flour
- 2 eggs
- 2 teaspoons baking powder

Directions:

1. Sift the flour, baking powder and salt in a container.
2. In a separate container, combine the butter and honey until fluffy. Stir in the eggs and vanilla and mix thoroughly.
3. Put in the flour mixture, alternating it with the milk.
4. Fold in the walnuts then spoon the batter in a 9-inch round cake pan coated with baking paper.
5. Pre-heat the oven and bake at 350F for about forty minutes or until it rises significantly and starts to appear golden-brown.
6. Let the cake cool in the pan and serve, sliced.

Nutritional Content of One Serving:
Calories: 351 | Fat: 18.5g | Protein: 7.6g | Carbohydrates: 42.1g

White Chocolate Blackberry Cake

Total Time Taken: 2 hours
Yield: 10 Servings
Ingredients:
Sponge cake:

- ¼ teaspoon salt
- ½ cup white sugar
- ½ teaspoon baking powder
- 1 cup all-purpose flour
- 5 eggs

Filling:

- 1 ½ cups heavy cream
- 2 ½ cups white chocolate chips
- 2 cups fresh blackberries

Directions:

1. For the sponge cake, whip the eggs, sugar and salt in a container until volume increases to twice what it was.
2. Fold in the flour and baking powder then spoon the batter in a 8-inch round cake pan coated with baking paper.
3. Pre-heat the oven and bake at 350F for around forty minutes then allow the cake to cool in the pan.
4. Slice the cake in half along the length.
5. For the filling, bring the cream to the boiling point in a saucepan. Turn off the heat and put in the chocolate. Stir until melted then let cool in your refrigerator.
6. Whip the white chocolate cream for at least two minutes until fluffy.
7. Fill the cake with half of the cream and half of the blackberries. Cover the cake with the rest of the cream and garnish with blackberries.
8. The cake tastes best chilled.

Nutritional Content of One Serving:
Calories: 418 | Fat: 22.8g | Protein: 7.3g | Carbohydrates: 48.3g

Whole Pear Sponge Cake

Total Time Taken: 2 hours
Yield: 14 Servings
Ingredients:

- ¼ cup canola oil
- ¼ cup honey
- ¼ teaspoon salt
- ½ cup butter, softened
- ½ cup cocoa powder
- ½ cup sour cream
- 1 ½ cups all-purpose flour
- 1 cinnamon stick
- 1 teaspoon baking soda
- 2 cups white wine
- 2 eggs
- 2 star anise
- 4 pears

Directions:

1. Peel the pears and place them in a saucepan. Put in the star anise, cinnamon, honey and wine and

cook over low heat for about half an hour. Let cool and then position the pears in a 9-inch round cake pan coated with baking paper.

2. Mix the butter, canola oil and eggs in a container until creamy.

3. Put in the sour cream and mix thoroughly then fold in the flour, cocoa powder, baking soda and salt.

4. Spoon the batter over the pears.

5. Preheat your oven and bake the cake for 45 minutes or until a toothpick inserted into the center of the cake comes out clean.

6. Let the cake cool before you serve.

Nutritional Content of One Serving:

Calories: 257 | Fat: 13.5g | Protein: 3.4g | Carbohydrates: 27.6g

Yeasted Plum Cake

Total Time Taken: 2 hours

Yield: 16 Servings

Ingredients:

- ¼ cup butter, melted
- ½ cup light brown sugar
- ½ cup warm milk
- ½ teaspoon salt
- 1 ¼ teaspoons instant yeast
- 1 cup warm water
- 1 pound plums, pitted and sliced
- 1 tablespoon lemon zest
- 1 teaspoon vanilla extract
- 2 eggs
- 3 cups all-purpose flour

Directions:

1. Mix the flour, salt and yeast in a container.
2. Put in the water, milk, butter, eggs, vanilla and lemon zest and knead the dough minimum ten minutes until it looks and feels elastic.
3. Allow the dough to rest for an hour then roll it into a rectangle and move it to a sheet cake pan coated with baking paper.
4. Top with plums and drizzle with brown sugar.
5. Pre-heat the oven and bake at 350F for about forty minutes or until it rises significantly and starts to appear golden-brown.
6. Let the cake cool in the pan before you serve.

Nutritional Content of One Serving:

Calories: 150 | Fat: 3.9g | Protein: 3.7g | Carbohydrates: 25.1g

Yogurt Bundt Cake

Total Time Taken: 1 ¼ hours

Yield: 12 Servings

Ingredients:

- ½ teaspoon salt
- 1 ½ cups plain yogurt
- 1 ½ cups white sugar
- 1 cup butter, softened
- 1 teaspoon baking powder
- 1 teaspoon baking soda
- 2 tablespoons lemon juice
- 2 tablespoons lemon zest
- 3 cups all-purpose flour
- 6 eggs, separated

Directions:

1. Mix the egg yolks with sugar until pale and fluffy. Stir in the butter and mix thoroughly.
2. Put in the lemon zest and juice then mix in the yogurt.
3. Fold in the flour, baking powder, baking soda and salt.
4. Spoon the batter in a greased Bundt cake pan and preheat your oven and bake at 350F for about forty minutes or until a toothpick inserted into the center of the cake comes out clean.
5. Let the cake cool in the pan before transferring on a platter.

Nutritional Content of One Serving:

Calories: 398 | Fat: 18.2g | Protein: 7.9g | Carbohydrates: 51.7g

Yogurt Strawberry Cake

Total Time Taken: 1 hour

Yield: 8 Servings

Ingredients:

- ½ cup cornstarch
- ½ teaspoon salt
- ¾ cup canola oil
- ¾ cup white sugar
- 1 ½ cups all-purpose flour
- 1 cup plain yogurt
- 1 cup strawberries, sliced
- 1 teaspoon baking powder
- 1 teaspoon vanilla extract
- 2 eggs

Directions:

1. Mix the canola oil, sugar, eggs and vanilla in a container until fluffy.
2. Stir in the yogurt and mix thoroughly then fold in the flour, cornstarch, baking powder and salt then pour the batter in a 9-inch round cake pan covered with parchment paper.
3. Top the cake with fresh strawberries and preheat your oven and bake at 350F for about forty minutes or until a toothpick inserted in the center comes out cleans.
4. Let the cake cool in the pan before you serve.

Nutritional Content of One Serving:

Calories: 412 | Fat: 22.2g | Protein: 5.7g | Carbohydrates: 47.9g

APPENDIX : RECIPES INDEX

Milton Keynes UK
Ingram Content Group UK Ltd.
UKHW030237171123
432716UK00001B/24

9 781802 440393